Your Family's Health

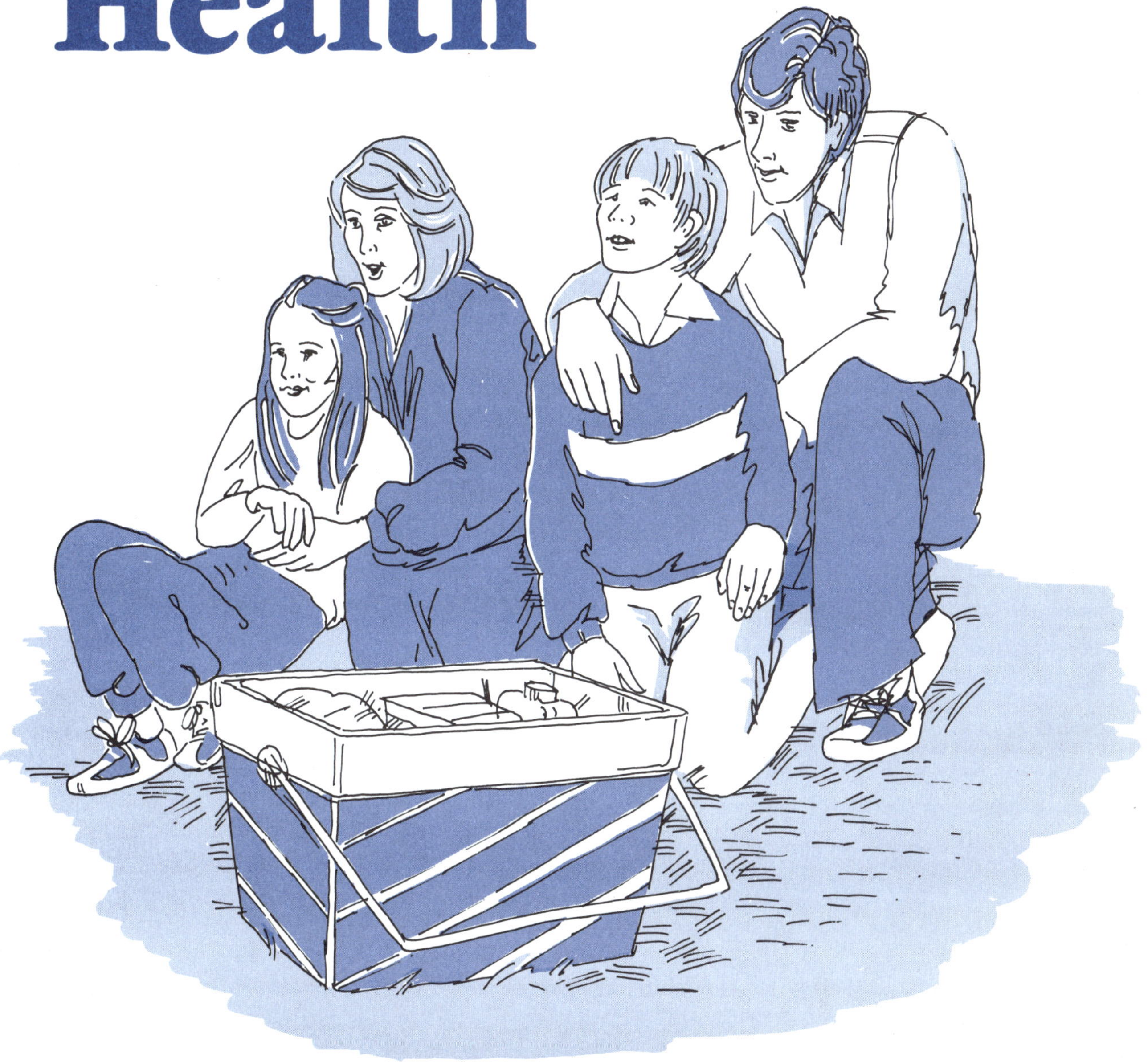

EDITORIAL
Managing Editor: Judy Poulos
Editor: Sheridan Carter
Editorial Coordinator: Margaret Kelly
Assistant Editors: Jutta Sieverding, Carol Galvin
UK Editor: Helen Travis
Sub Editor: Ella Martin

ILLUSTRATIONS
Carol Dunn

PRODUCTION
Tara Barrett
Chris Hatcher

COVER DESIGN
Design: Nadia Sbisa
Photography: Harm Mol
Chair supplied by Freedom Furniture, Surry Hills, NSW

DESIGN AND PRODUCTION MANAGER
Nadia Sbisa

PUBLISHER
Philippa Sandall

YOUR FAMILY'S HEALTH
Includes Index
ISBN 1 86343 025 3

Family Circle is a registered trademark of IPC Magazines Ltd.
Published by J.B. Fairfax Press Ltd by arrangement with IPC Magazines Ltd.

Formatted by J.B. Fairfax Press Pty Ltd
Output by Adtype, Sydney
Printed by Toppan Printing Co, Hong Kong

Distributed by J.B. Fairfax Press Ltd
9 Trinity Centre, Park Farm Estate
Wellingborough, Northants
Telephone: (0933) 402330
Facsimile: (0933) 402234

CONTENTS

Acknowledgments
I would like to thank my family who have always supported my endeavours;
from birth on my parents, my grandparents and, a little later, my brother and for the last twenty years my husband, John, and his parents and more recently, my son.
My thanks also to my colleague Doctor Gwenyth Francis for her helpful review of this book.
Thanks also to the staff of J.B. Fairfax Press who, under the able direction of Philippa Sandall, have transformed my scribblings into a book.

INTRODUCTION

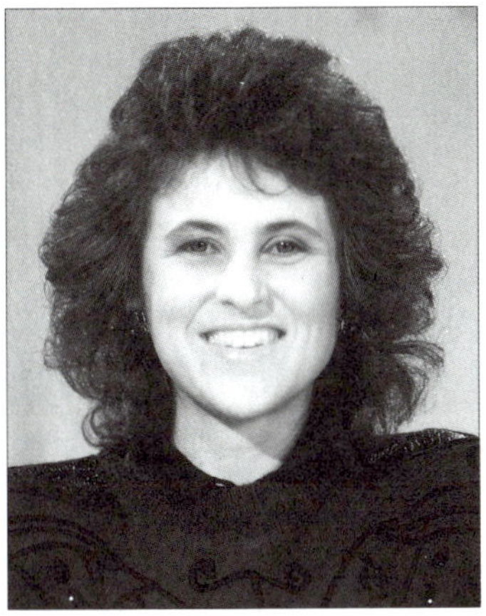

This book was written to cover many of the questions that people ask me, either in my surgery or in my weekly magazine column. After spending ten years as a columnist, as well as some time on radio and television, I think I'm aware of many of the 'grass roots' medical issues that really worry people.

My aim is to arm you with the confidence and the questions you may need to get the most out of a consultation with your doctor. I see this book as providing a resource for you to use as you need. Having been a patient, as well as a doctor, I try not to lose sight of the fact that being a patient is often worrying. When people enter a doctor's surgery they carry anxiety about their symptoms as well as anxiety and embarrassment about how their problem will be received by that other human being, the doctor. These anxieties can make it difficult to remember what you have been told about your condition. With this in mind, I hope you will use this book to gain information, even as a checklist, which will allow you to get the most out of your consultation with your doctor.

I am very interested in improving my communication on health issues. My own career seems to have developed in three strands – all concerned with this communication. Firstly, there is my work in my own general practice. Secondly, there is my work in the media. The third strand involves teaching doctors about general practice. In all three areas I constantly strive to improve my understanding of the most worthwhile medical information that needs to be considered.

Dr Fran was born in Sydney, Australia. Apart from her medical degree, she also has an Arts degree. She has worked in general practice for nearly fifteen years. For twelve years Dr Fran has been involved in teaching other doctors. She has written a weekly magazine column for about eight years and has made regular appearances on radio and television. Married to John for nearly twenty years, they have one delightful seven-year-old son, Nicholas. She lists her interests as sailing, skiing, tennis, swimming, ice skating, dancing, reading, theatre, good food, writing, conversation and holidays.

HEALTH & DIET

Good nutrition is vital to your overall health and wellbeing. Today, many of the diseases associated with lifestyle, such as coronary disease, high blood pressure and some cancers, are increasing because people are ignoring basic good health guidelines.

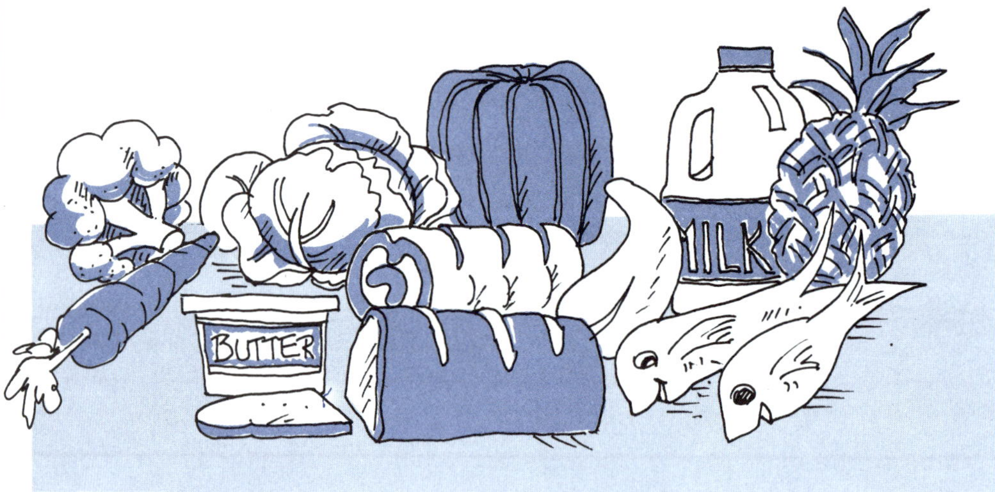

Good health guidelines

What can you do to help keep yourself healthy?
The answer is simple. Reduce the risk factors that cause lifestyle disease. All it takes is the willpower to follow these basic guidelines for good health.

- ❑ A well-balanced diet to maintain a healthy weight
- ❑ Regular exercise, suitable to your age and fitness
- ❑ Adequate sleep
- ❑ Time for relaxation including regular holidays
- ❑ No smoking or other nonprescribed drugs
- ❑ No alcohol or only in moderation
- ❑ Reduced caffeine intake

Many of the risk factors associated with disease today arise because people are so used to 'immediate gratification' that they rely on fast food outlets when they are hungry and take pills when unwell, rather than change their lifestyle.

A balanced diet

In ages past, people were at risk of undernutrition – we are at risk because of the opposite. Not only do we eat too much of the wrong foods but our diet includes a lot of highly processed and refined foods, lacking in dietary fibre.

Good nutrition is vital to overall health and wellbeing. The Healthy Diet Pyramid shows how you can quite easily achieve a balanced diet and maintain your appropriate weight.

Eat most foods

These are the foods that are low in fat and rich in dietary fibre.

❑ ***Bread and cereals*** (preferably wholegrain) are a good source of B complex vitamins, particularly thiamine (B1).

❑ ***Vegetables and fruits*** (including fresh, frozen, dried and canned) are a good source of vitamin C and the yellow, orange and green varieties are rich in vitamin A. Vegetables should include legumes or pulses such as dried peas, beans and lentils, including canned baked beans, kidney beans and bean mixes.

NUTRITION TIPS

- ❑ Eat a variety of foods
- ❑ Eat more bread, cereal, fruit and vegetables
- ❑ Eat less fat
- ❑ Eat less sugar
- ❑ Eat less salt

Eat moderately foods

These are the foods that are rich in protein, necessary for the growth and repair of all tissues and a good source of the B complex vitamins.

❑ ***Lean meat, poultry (no skin), fish, eggs and nuts*** If you want to reduce your blood cholesterol level as well, remove all visible fat and prepare food with little or no fat.

❑ ***Milk, cheese and yoghurt*** You should use the reduced and low-fat varieties for adults and children from school age onwards after checking with your doctor. During their first two years, children need whole milk to get sufficient kilojoules (calories) for growth.

Eat in small amounts foods

❑ ***Margarine and reduced-fat spreads*** (including the polyunsaturated varieties).

❑ ***Butter and oil*** (including mono-unsaturates) such as olive, canola, peanut and the polyunsaturated oils.

❑ ***Sugar and sugar-based foods*** such as confectionery, jam and soft drinks. Children see these foods advertised incessantly and want them. It is often hard to resist their demands but when it comes to obesity, prevention is better than cure.

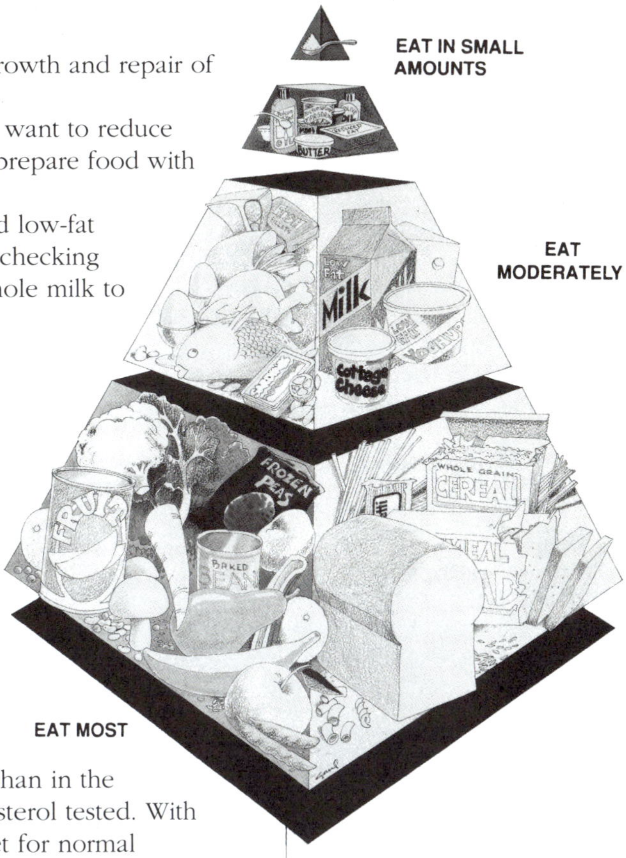

The Healthy Diet Pyramid and text by courtesy of the Australian Nutrition Foundation

Cholesterol

Many more people seem to have cholesterol-related problems than in the past. This is partly because more people are having their cholesterol tested. With increased research into heart disease, lower limits have been set for normal cholesterol. A much larger number of people are now classified as having a high cholesterol level.

Premenopausal women have some protection against heart disease due to a hormonal effect, which is lost as they become menopausal.

People need to be individually assessed when cholesterol levels are too high. Although a high cholesterol level is one of the major factors associated with coronary artery disease, it is not the only one. A family history of heart disease, smoking, increased blood pressure and diabetes also contribute.

❑ ***What can you do to lower your cholesterol?*** Paying attention to your diet and lowering the amount of cholesterol you eat, can work wonders for most people. If your cholesterol is not lowered by diet alone, your doctor may prescribe appropriate medication as well.

Fibre

There is an emphasis today on encouraging people to eat more high-fibre foods. A high-fibre diet encourages normal bowel function, and may prevent a number of diseases that seem to be related to a diet high in cholesterol and fats. A healthy diet should include a range of fibre-rich foods. Simply adding unprocessed bran or oat bran to your ordinary diet, does not bring all the benefits of fibre.

FIBRE FACTS

❑ Fibre is nature's 'appetite suppressant' and bulking agent

❑ It helps promote bowel regularity

❑ Soluble fibre which is found in oats and some other foods can help remove cholesterol from the blood

Low blood sugar

Low blood sugar (hypoglycaemia) is a rare medical condition. Nonmedical health practitioners sometimes diagnose low blood sugar more often than the rate at which it is known medically to occur. The diagnosis of true hypoglycaemia can easily be made by medically analysing a series of blood samples.

An unfounded diagnosis of hypoglycaemia is often made by nonmedical practitioners when people complain of feeling chronically tired, anxious, depressed and unable to cope. This is often not correct and other causes for the symptoms should be investigated. High blood sugar (diabetes mellitus), commonly abbreviated to diabetes, is more common.

HEALTH & DIET

As well as the physical health risks, being overweight can lower your confidence and self esteem

What is a healthy weight?

Overweight people have a higher incidence of high blood pressure, high blood fats, heart disease, diabetes and gall bladder disease than the rest of the population. Too much or too little weight can affect how your body functions and how you feel about yourself. There is no such thing as a single ideal weight for any height but there is a healthy weight range, based on a Body Mass Index (BMI) which measures body fat in adults. You can work out your BMI by dividing your weight in kilograms by the square of your height in metres. Your BMI should be between 20 and 25.

Obesity

It is true that 'fatness runs in families' but this does not mean you have to be fat just because your parents were. Take it as a warning that you have to take care.

Overweight people are faced with a huge choice of diets. Some 'magic' diets claim that you can lose weight without effort but the truth is that most of these 'fad' diets result in very short-term weight loss. The only lasting answer to obesity is to establish healthy eating patterns that you can stick to forever, and a sensible exercise program. This means a change in your eating behaviour. Weight loss is like the tortoise, slow and steady. You only gain weight if the kilojoules (calories) provided by the food you take in, exceed the kilojoules your body uses up. Combining a low-kilojoule intake diet with increased exercise will achieve results.

Some people find they benefit by attending a support group. Others can accomplish sensible weight loss alone or under the supervision of their doctor or a dietitian. One very successful method is to keep a food diary, and use a reward system (not food) to encourage yourself. It is also important to identify your own personal danger times for overeating and think of strategies to overcome them. Instead of eating, go for a walk, phone a friend, or give yourself a treat.

❑ ***Can surgery help?*** You should only contemplate surgery if you are very, very obese. Before undergoing such a procedure, you will need to be properly assessed. You should be told of the side effects and any other risks. Do not take this decision lightly. So many people, who are only a little or moderately overweight, see surgery as an easy way out. It is not. Losing weight involves accepting that you are overweight and being motivated enough to change your eating and exercise patterns for life! Others can encourage and help you, but no-one else can do it for you.

TRUE OR FALSE?

❑ *Only teenage girls have eating disorders.*
False

❑ *If you have an eating disorder you must be thin.*
False. Many average-size and overweight people have grossly abnormal eating patterns

Eating disorders

The first sign of an eating disorder is often an intense interest in food and weight. It can be hard to pick up these early signs. People with eating disorders often find it very difficult to discuss the problem. They try to keep it secret and often experience anxiety, depression and social withdrawal because of their need to hide the problem. People suffering from an eating disorder can often be helped by special programs, designed to help them alter their behaviour.

❑ **Anorexia nervosa** starts with wanting to lose weight. Sufferers become extremely thin, but still see themselves as being fat. Their body size may become so reduced that complications develop. They eat very little and combine this with excessive exercising. Menstruation may stop once a girl or woman's weight falls below a certain level. Some sufferers may overeat then induce vomiting or use laxatives to stop food being absorbed

❑ **Bulimia nervosa** This condition is characterised by the consumption of huge amounts of food in so-called 'eating binges', followed by self-induced vomiting or laxative use. Unlike the anorexic, the bulimic person may maintain a near-normal body weight. It is the total preoccupation with weight and diet coupled with the abnormal behaviour to maintain the weight that distinguishes the disease.

❑ **Compulsive eating** concerns the obese person who binges. Compulsive eaters don't use purgatives or vomiting so they rapidly become overweight. These people are characterised by frequent attempts to lose weight – without success. Their weight fluctuates and they are in danger of developing the medical complications of being obese.

HEIGHT AND WEIGHT CHARTS

These healthy weight ranges are based on data from a number of studies which show acceptable weights consistent with lowest mortality (from Garrow, 1981, *Classification of Obesity*, Churchill Livingstone).

FOR WOMEN AND MEN 18 YEARS UPWARDS

Height (without shoes)			Body Weight (in light clothing without shoes)
140 cm	4 ft	7 ins	39 - 40 kg
142	4	8	40 - 50
144	4	9	41 - 52
146	4	9½	43 - 53
148	4	10	44 - 55
150	4	11	45 - 56
152	5	0	46 - 58
154	5	1	47 - 59
156	5	1½	49 - 61
158	5	2	50 - 62
160	5	3	51 - 64
162	5	4	52 - 66
164	5	4½	54 - 67
166	5	5	55 - 69
168	5	6	56 - 71
170	5	7	58 - 72
172	5	8	59 - 74
174	5	8½	61 - 76
176	5	9	62 - 77
178	5	10	63 - 79
180	5	11	65 - 81
182	6	0	66 - 83
184	6	½	68 - 85
186	6	1	69 - 86
188	6	2	71 - 88
190	6	3	72 - 90
192	6	4	74 - 92
194	6	4½	75 - 94
196	6	5	77 - 96
198	6	6	78 - 98
200	6	7	80 - 100

METRIC CONVERTER

kg	st	lb
1.0	0	2
6.4	1	0
10	1	8
20	3	2
40	6	4
44	6	13
46	7	4
48	7	8
50	7	13
52	8	3
54	8	7
56	8	12
58	9	2
60	9	6
62	9	11
64	10	2
66	10	6
68	10	10
70	11	1
72	11	5
74	11	10
76	12	0
78	12	4
80	12	9
82	12	13
84	13	4
86	13	8
88	13	13
90	14	0
92	14	4
95	14	11
100	15	8
127	20	0

EXERCISE FACTS

- If starting an exercise from scratch, be careful not to do too much too soon
- Don't keep exercising through an illness
- If you stop your exercise program, restart slowly
- Don't exercise on a full stomach
- Use the correct equipment, including shoes
- Choose an exercise that suits your age and fitness

LOSE WEIGHT ACTION PLAN

- Set realistic short-term and long-term goals
- Follow the Healthy Pyramid guidelines
- Keep all meals and snacks low in fat and sugar
- Drink alcohol only moderately or not at all
- Do some regular exercise
- Drink more water

Regular exercise

The current interest in exercise and the desire for fitness is a positive and healthy trend. However, like all fashion it can be excessive. During exercise, chemical substances called endorphins, which act like naturally occurring opiates, can be released. You can become high on exercise. This is why exercise can be helpful if you are feeling down. Some people become obsessive and exercise through illnesses. This is one explanation of the rare deaths that occur in fit young people.

KILOJOULE BURNERS

Light 10-20 kJ (2-5 cals) burned per minute	**Moderate** 20-30 kJ (5-8 cals) burned per minute	**Heavy** 30-40 kJ (8-10 cals) burned per minute	**Very Heavy** over 40 kJ (10 cals) burned per minute
Walking, slow	Walking, fast	Jogging	Swimming, training
Bowling, lawn or ten pin	Gardening, heavy	Skipping	Squash, advanced
Golf	Tennis	Country dancing	Cross-country skiing
Table tennis	Bicycling	Disco dancing	Marathon running
Housework, light	Horseriding	Aerobics	Rowing
Gardening, light	Skating	Downhill skiing	Basketball
Yoga	Swimming, moderate	Netball	Uphill hiking
Water skiing	Ballroom dancing	Football	Fast bicycling
Painting	Sailing	Hockey	
Carpentry	Surfing	Climbing stairs	
Light industry	Hiking		
Assembly work			
Clerical work			

Courtesy of the Australian Nutrition Foundation

Other exercise-induced injuries involve overuse syndromes in which a particular muscle or ligament is used so often that symptoms develop. Although regular exercise is desirable from a health point of view, it should be undertaken in a sensible manner so as to reap its benefits.

If you feel you have no time to exercise, take a closer look at your lifestyle. Often it is not a lack of time so much as your priorities or inclination that stand in the way. If you have not been exercising and would like to do so, discuss your exercise plans with your doctor. Exercise burns up kilojoules and raises your body's metabolic rate. Find an exercise that suits your lifestyle and do it regularly.

Relaxation

In today's pressured society, it is appropriate for all of us to be able to use a self-relaxation technique. There are many variations of basically the same technique. All involve progressively learning to relax the muscles of your body and then to concentrate on relaxing your mind.

Lie flat and, starting at your head, release all the tension in your muscles, temples, jaw and so on down your whole body. Concentrate on each area separately, relaxing shoulders, arms, abdomen, until you reach your toes. At the same time relax your mind by imagining a pastoral scene or a flower, or concentrating on a sound or word. Different methods will appeal to different people.

- ***Holidays*** Your life should include time to indulge in relaxing healthy activities. Many people push themselves and often ignore the need for regular holidays. Everyone needs a break. Some people need to physically change their environment in order to switch off.

If it is difficult for you to take holidays, then set priorities in your life. Learn to say no. Change goals, and jobs if necessary, so you won't find yourself caught in a rut.

Adequate sleep

There is a great variation in the amount of sleep that different people need. Some function well on as little as five or six hours, others require nine to ten hours. If you are anxious or depressed, your sleep may well be disturbed. Laboratory studies in which sleeping is monitored for a night have shown that many people, particularly those describing themselves as insomniacs, sleep more than they think.

If you wake during the night and can't get back to sleep, get up and do something else for a while, such as ironing, reading or watching television. Bed should only be associated with two activities – sleeping and sex.

❑ ***Sleeping tablet addiction*** Avoid long-term sleeping medications. If you become addicted to sleeping tablets, do not stop suddenly. Sleeping tablets and tranquillising drugs must be stopped gradually, under medical supervision.

Noise can affect the quality of sleep. If you are in a noisy environment, try to block out the noise by sound-proofing, concealing it beneath a constant level of sound, such as an air-conditioner or resorting to ear plugs.

WHAT CAN YOU DO TO HELP YOURSELF SLEEP?

- ❑ Relax before going to bed, perhaps by having a warm bath
- ❑ Avoid exercising just before going to bed. It can have a stimulating effect
- ❑ Avoid caffeine-containing substances in the latter half of the day
- ❑ A glass of warm milk can decrease your level of arousal and help you sleep
- ❑ Learn a relaxation technique that will help you relax during the day and fall asleep at night
- ❑ Don't sleep in to make up for lost sleep during the night. It is better to go to bed later in a more tired state

Smoking and health

If you are a smoker who would like to give it up, there are programs designed to help you. Your family doctor may run one or may be able to direct you to one. The health risks of smoking include strokes, cancer and inflammation of the respiratory tract, heart attacks, stomach, cervical and urinary cancer and circulatory problems. There are also a number of unattractive cosmetic effects of smoking, such as bad breath and dull skin. Wrinkles form prematurely round the eyes and mouth, and spots and blemishes can develop because of reduced oxygen in the blood. Your teeth become stained and your hair and clothes smell.

Nicotine chewing gum has a place in helping you get over the withdrawal symptoms, but it is only a temporary measure and is not a substitute for cigarettes. Only you can decide to become a nonsmoker and only you can make it happen.

Alcohol

Alcohol, like smoking, can damage many different parts of your body including brain, liver and kidneys. The misuse of alcohol is responsible for many so-called minor health problems, such as tiredness, poor concentration, indigestion and insomnia. It is also associated with major problems in our society including road accidents, marital and family distress, violent crime and work problems.

Many people underestimate their drinking and do not associate their symptoms or social difficulties with a drinking problem. They react to a comment that they are drinking too much by pointing out it is 'social drinking' and that their friends drink as much or more than they do. People suffering from alcohol related problems will often deny the problem and become angry when questioned by family, friends or employers. Signs that alcohol consumption has reached problem level include a change in drinking habits, episodes of memory loss and problems with jobs, marriage or family.

How much alcohol is safe for adults?

- ❑ Women: Up to one or two standard drinks four or five times weekly.
- ❑ Men: Up to three or four standard drinks four or five times weekly.

WHAT IS A STANDARD DRINK?

30 mL (1 oz) spirits
285 mL (10 oz) beer
120 mL (4 oz) wine
60 mL (2 oz) fortified wine
570 mL (20 oz) low alcohol beer

You and your doctor

CHOOSING A DOCTOR

Some factors to consider when choosing your doctor are:

- ❑ Accessibility
- ❑ Continuity
- ❑ Compatibility

Which doctor?

General practitioners are also known as 'family doctors'. Family doctors expect to give continuity of care over a period of time. The recording of notes and medical histories means that if you need to see another member of the practice, or a locum, he or she should be able to continue your treatment. The advantage of attending a particular doctor or practice is that you should be able to expect total ongoing care.

Some forms of medical care are 'episodic', which means that you may go to a different doctor each time you are sick. The disadvantage of this is that important links between different episodes of illness may be missed.

❑ ***Referrals*** You can expect that your family doctor will treat you to the best of his or her knowledge or seek out more specialised help if necessary. It may involve referring you to an appropriate specialist, even organising the appointment for you if it is urgent. Your family doctor is your advocate. Getting you into hospital or to see a particular specialist is not always easy. Not every referral will have a satisfactory outcome. If you are not satisfied, ask for a 'second opinion'. Give your family doctor both good and bad feedback on referrals for future reference.

❑ ***Visiting your doctor*** First of all, your doctor will ask about your medical history. The next steps are determined by what your history has revealed. Your doctor will make a decision as to whether, and what kind of physical examination need be undertaken and whether any tests need to be requested.

Your doctor should give you an explanation of your situation, and together you should agree on a plan of action. The concept of working together is very important and this is why you need to choose a doctor with whom you feel comfortable and able to talk.

❑ ***When to see your doctor*** You should feel happy about seeing your doctor whenever you are worried about a problem. Too many people hold back from going to their doctor with complaints which they regard as too trivial, or too embarrassing to discuss. Many become seriously ill as a result. Often communicating the problem and having the doctor's reassurance that you are not alone, can be of enormous benefit. After all, a large part of a family doctor's job is reassurance and education.

Don't ignore fairly major symptoms and wait until disease is well advanced before seeking help. Prevention is better than cure and you may be in much more trouble if you wait

The medical check-up

Adults should be checked regularly for blood pressure, cholesterol, blood fats, urine and weight. Women need regular breast checks, cervical/PAP smear tests and pelvic examinations. Men need regular prostate and testicle checks. Your doctor can advise on the frequency of diabetes screening and any other tests you may need, according to your personal risk factors and family and personal medical history.

HOME MONITORING CHRONIC ILLNESSES

Today many chronic illnesses can be well managed at home, with the patient playing a more active part in monitoring and understanding the disease.

Diabetics can	❑ test own urine ❑ use blood glucose machines ❑ administer own injections
Asthmatics can	❑ monitor airflow by measuring airflow rates ❑ manage own drugs
Hypertensives can	❑ monitor fluctuating blood pressure (performed with a device that gives a digital readout)
Obese people can	❑ monitor weight (see Section on eating disorders)

COMMON INVESTIGATIONS

Barium enema

This is a special type of X-ray to look at the bowel. Barium is inserted with an enema into your rectum after the bowel has been adequately cleared. The barium coats the bowel so that the X-ray shows its outline. In this way, growths such as polyps and tumours can be identified. Diverticula, small pocketings in the intestine, can also be detected.

Barium meal

This investigation applies the same principle as barium enema to study the stomach and upper bowel and to pick up peptic ulcers or cancers.

Blood tests

There are different blood tests for different purposes. Some are diagnostic, others monitor changes. Blood grouping is often required during pregnancy and before major surgery. Blood tests may be repeated to check on the progress of treatment.

Bronchoscopy

In this test, an instrument is passed through the mouth or nose into the air passages. It allows the lining of the air passages and lungs to be seen. Specimens can be taken for microscopic examination in the diagnosis of cancer and infection.

CAT scan

A new type of X-ray first developed for evaluating the brain, but is now used for the whole body. Multiple X-rays are taken at different angles and analysed by the computer. While the cost of these CAT scans is high, this technique means that more invasive and potentially harmful procedures are used less often.

Chest X-ray

This provides information about the lungs, heart, major blood vessels in your chest and the surrounding bony cage. A chest X-ray may be ordered if an infection, cancer or any other lung disease is suspected, or if some structural problem such as a broken rib is suspected. The chest X-ray can also detect heart enlargement.

Cystoscopy

This test involves passing a tube through the urethra into the bladder. Sometimes dye may also be introduced and followed by X-rays. This is not only a way of looking at kidney and bladder function but polyps may be removed or inflamed areas treated by heat, through the cystoscope.

Electrocardiogram (ECG)

Electrodes are placed on various parts of your chest. The leads attached to the electrodes record the electrical changes that occur in your heart. This type of test can pick up an irregular heartbeat.

There are a number of different types of irregularity, each giving off a characteristic waveform. A heart attack causes damage to the heart muscle which is reflected in electrical changes, picked up on ECG tracing.

You may be surprised to learn that the patient is not always aware that a heart attack has occurred. Evidence of the occurrence may only be picked up on an ECG tracing.

Exercise or stress ECG

This type of ECG takes a recording while you are doing exercises which place some stress on the heart. Sometimes the effects of narrowed arteries (coronary artery disease) are not seen on a resting ECG. The stress or exercise ECG may pick up significant changes.

Continuous ECG

A 24-hour Holter monitor provides a continuous ECG recording over twenty-four hours. Sometimes people may notice that their heart beats irregularly, but when they attend a doctor, their heart rate and rhythm is normal. A 24-hour ECG may help pick up these irregularities as well as indicate the occurrence of silent heart attacks. The test may need to be repeated to get a result.

Endoscopy, gastroscopy and colonoscopy

These three investigations all use the same principle of passing a tube into a particular part of the gastrointestinal tract. The first two methods involve passing the tube through the oesophagus, whereas colonoscopy involves passing the tube through the rectum. These tests allow the doctor direct visualisation as well as the opportunity to sample and photograph the areas of gut being investigated. The procedure is usually done under local anaesthesia and a muscle relaxant is also often used.

Lung function tests

These tests help to assess how well your lungs are working. Many people with asthma and chronic bronchitis have peak flowmeters to assess their lung functions.

Ultrasound

This procedure involves obtaining an image of an organ by using high frequency sound waves. The procedure is often used in pregnancy, as it provides an outline of the developing fetus and placenta within the uterus. The procedure is painless but because the pelvic ultrasound requires a full bladder, it can be a little uncomfortable. The procedure is generally regarded as harmless. An abdominal ultrasound may now also be ordered, to look for gall stones, perhaps making more invasive methods of diagnosis unnecessary.

HEALTH MATTERS

You strive for good health but from time to time you will have to deal with the symptoms of illness and the results of accidents. Knowing what you can do yourself, when to ask for help and how to find it can certainly limit disability and even save lives.

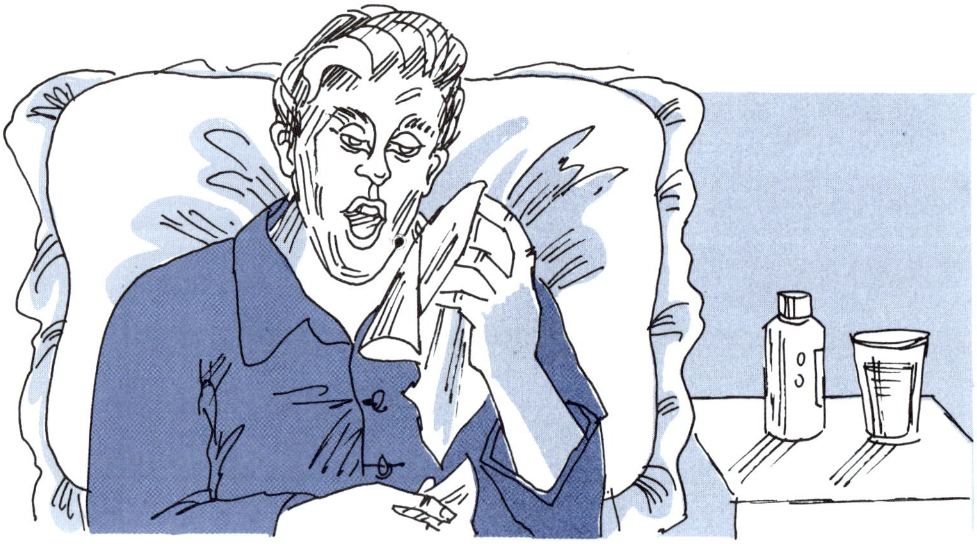

Common symptoms

Coughs

Your doctor will want to know where you think the cough is coming from, how long it has been present and if you are coughing up mucus (if so what colour and is there any blood in it). You should also mention any other symptoms such as chest pain, fever and breathlessness.

Dry throat coughs, associated with inflammation or irritation above the voice box or larynx, are best helped by sucking and chewing lozenges. A cough suppressant may help a dry, irritating cough which originates lower than the larynx. Do not take these for more than a few days without checking with your doctor.

A productive cough may well need antibiotics. A simple expectorant is often helpful but it may cause you to vomit or have painful stomach cramps. Most importantly, remember that warm drinks and steam inhalations will help all types of cough. Anyone with a cough should stop smoking and avoid others who smoke.

Headache

This common symptom is rarely due to serious and dangerous causes. Having said that, however, any new, severe or sudden headache warrants a medical consultation. Headaches may be due to any one of a number of common causes, some of which are discussed below. Tension headaches are a common cause of recurring headache, due to muscle spasm in the head and neck.

❑ ***Migraine*** Migraine can present in a number of different ways. It runs in families and is more common in women than in men. It is often associated with nausea and vomiting. Migraine is often preceded by an 'aura', usually a visual one, in which stars, jagged or flashing lights are seen. The headache is usually on one side.

There are a number of different drugs available to try to prevent frequent migraine or to treat the occasional one. The usual approach is to try a particular medication, moving on to others if this does not work. Treatment may require a medication to help empty the stomach as migraine delays this process, making it difficult to absorb pain-relief medication. Analgesics, combined with rest in a darkened room, are often effective. In rare cases, severe migraine can become a debilitating condition.

❑ ***Sinusitis*** Sinusitis is another common form of headache, diagnosed by tenderness over the sinuses. This type of headache is made worse by movement and bending. Steam inhalation and nasal sniffing of clean salt water can help clear the sinuses. Antibiotics will be prescribed if an infection is thought to be present. If you also suffer from an allergy, antihistamines and special nasal sprays will be tried.

❑ ***High blood pressure*** How often high blood pressure results in headaches is still debatable. There is the rare patient who can anticipate a rise in blood pressure because of a headache. However, a great many people cannot judge their blood pressure reading by how they are feeling. Many people who have high blood pressure develop headaches when their blood pressure is normal. It is usual for a doctor to check your blood pressure if you come in with a headache.

❑ ***Other causes*** More serious causes of headache include infections, such as meningitis and encephalitis, brain tumours and bleeding into the brain area.

WHEN SHOULD YOU SEE YOUR DOCTOR?

See your doctor if you have:

- ❑ headache, accompanied by a fever and stiff neck
- ❑ sudden onset of headache
- ❑ a change in pattern of headache in chronic headache sufferer
- ❑ headache associated with visual difficulties or neurological problems
- ❑ headache associated with head injury
- ❑ persistent headache
- ❑ headaches that worsen in the morning or wake you up

To diagnose your headache, the doctor will take your history, examine your neck, head, eyes, ears, jaw and teeth and measure your blood pressure. Lifestyle is very important in dealing with chronic headache. Learning and using relaxation techniques and stress avoidance can be very beneficial. Your doctor may be able to assist by showing you relaxation techniques, or by directing you to community resources where they can be learned

Weight loss

Unexplained weight loss, not related to dieting, must be taken seriously. It can be a sign of some underlying disorder, not apparently related to diet. Your doctor will look for emotional problems including depression, eating disorders, overactivity of the thyroid gland, cancer, chronic disease, chronic infection or the side-effect of medications that can decrease appetite, particularly in the elderly.

Accidents

One of the most frequent health problems you will need to cope with is the result of accidents, particularly those occurring around your own home.

Burns

Treat burns immediately by applying cold water to the affected area for ten to thirty minutes. Don't use ice as this can stick to the fragile burnt skin and rip it off. Don't burst blisters. Don't apply pressure to burnt skin or remove clothing that has become attached to the burn. You can cover badly burned areas with a bandage. A clean sheet or pillowcase is a useful bandage for a large burn if nothing else is available. Give adequate pain relief and maintain strictly antiseptic conditions, as infection can easily develop in burn areas. See a doctor or casualty department for assessment as soon as possible.

TENSION HEADACHES

❑ Often associated with increasing bouts of migraine

❑ Muscles of the neck and jaw contract

❑ Treatment can be by oral medication, physiotherapy, relaxation techniques and reducing stress factors in lifestyle

In an emergency, time is precious. To avoid panic it is useful to have an emergency plan. Give some thought to what you should do in a crisis, whom you should contact and where you should go

Cuts

Most cuts affect only the skin and underlying fatty tissue. Immediate treatment is to clean well with soap and water and apply antiseptic. If foreign material, such as dirt or glass, remains in the wound, you will need help from your doctor to remove it. If you are sure that stitching is not required, dry the cleansed wound and use butterfly plasters to draw the wound edges together. If stitching is required, it should be done within eight hours. If the wound is left, bacteria can enter and become trapped, making stitching undesirable. You may also require a tetanus injection.

Puncture wounds caused by sharp objects, including nails, pins and tacks, are generally regarded as trivial but should be treated with respect. Infection can easily be introduced under the skin by dirty objects and damage to blood vessels, nerves and tendons may occur. Signs of infection, such as swelling, fever and redness, can take a day or so to develop and a tetanus injection may be needed. Puncture wounds from instruments under pressure can result in severe damage to the underlying tissue so a doctor *must* be consulted.

Immediate treatment of puncture wounds involves cleaning to prevent infection. Soaking the wound in warm water for a few minutes twice over the next two days will help keep the puncture open, encouraging drainage and preventing infection. Your doctor will decide whether the wound requires further exploration or can be treated at home, or whether antibiotics are necessary.

All cuts, other than the obviously trivial ones, should be assessed medically. Depending on the area affected, your doctor will check that the underlying structures have not been seriously damaged. He will also need to assess whether stitching the wound is necessary.

Bites and stings

Bites from poisonous creatures need immediate action. Bites or stings from known nonpoisonous or noninfected animals require cooling and antiseptic cream. Sometimes an allergic reaction can develop which varies from mild swelling and itchiness to life-threatening breathing problems. Get medical help as soon as possible if swelling around the throat and face results in breathing problems. In milder forms of swelling and itching an antihistamine may be prescribed.

People who know they are allergic to a particular sting, for example a bee or wasp sting, may well have been advised as to the emergency medication they are required to take, and fast action may be needed to administer that treatment. Seek urgent medical care if an allergic reaction occurs, or if the person is in a state of shock. Support the breathing, if necessary, by using expired air resuscitation, also commonly known as mouth to mouth (see more on this technique on page 19). Use external cardiac massage as well as expired air resuscitation if the heart has stopped.

Pressure immobilisation is a technique of bandaging used to prevent the poison entering the bloodstream. It involves applying pressure to the bitten area and bandaging the whole limb. In the case of a bite by a poisonous animal or insect, you will need to take the victim to medical help as soon as possible where an anti-venene may be available.

In the case of a sting, remove the sting by scraping it out. Don't squeeze or pull the poison sac. Clean the wound and apply ice.

IF A TOOTH IS KNOCKED OUT

- ❑ Don't let it dry out
- ❑ Don't scrape or rub it
- ❑ Don't rinse in water for long
- ❑ Don't use antiseptics

See the dentist quickly

Tooth avulsion

The earlier a tooth is replanted in the gum, the better – ideally within thirty minutes. There is something you can do while waiting for the dentist. Hold the tooth only by the crown and don't touch the root. If the tooth is clean, replace it in the gum and hold it there with a finger or with aluminium foil moulded over the tooth and surrounding teeth. Even if the root appears broken, replace it in its socket. If the tooth is dirty, rinse it in milk and then replant. If milk is unavailable, use normal saline (salt solution), the patient's saliva or rinse it briefly under the tap and then replant it. If you cannot replant the tooth, cover it in milk or saline or cover it in plastic kitchen wrap while you take it to the dentist.

Sprains and strains

Sprains affect the ligaments, which are the tissues connecting bones on one side of the joint to the other. The knee and ankle are two common joints in which sprains occur. A ligamentous strain refers to the part of the ligament becoming stretched. A ligamentous sprain means that the ligament is partly torn at the ends. A torn ligament means that the ligament is no longer attached to one of the bones. Sometimes the ligament takes a fragment of bone with it, causing a fracture.

The basic home treatment for ligamentous injuries is to rest the injured part, apply ice or a cold pack regularly during the first twenty-four to thirty-six hours, use a compression bandage and elevate the affected part.

A torn ligament requires surgical attention. X-rays are used in more severe injuries to detect fractures but will not show up a partially torn ligament, which your doctor will diagnose on examination. A rehabilitation program, involving physiotherapy and muscle-strengthening exercises, will help to restore fitness.

R. I. C. E

R.I.C.E will help you remember what to do with sprains and strains

R = Rest
I = Ice
C = Compression
E = Elevation

Breaks

It is not always possible to tell if a bone has been broken just by looking. When a broken bone is suspected, an X-ray will be taken. Many fractured bones are in a good position for healing to take place. If not, they will need to be manipulated into the correct position and a cast applied to keep the bone fragments stable and to stop them moving about. Your body then heals the break. Sometimes bones are fractured in such a way that they require stabilisation from within, using pins and plates to hold the bones together. Fractured bones can affect neighbouring nerves and blood vessels. If you suspect a fracture may be present, see your doctor.

Head injury

Head injuries can be serious. Fortunately the contents of the head are well protected so that minor bumps should not cause injury. Problems following head injury may take time to appear so it is a good idea to observe the injured person for forty-eight hours after the injury. The changes to look for include persistent headache, vomiting, bleeding or fluid from ears, eyes and mouth. In addition, there may be changes in behaviour, including excessive sleepiness and tiredness. Call for immediate help if the pupils appear unequal. Ask your doctor if you are in doubt.

Poisoning

Poisons can be swallowed, inhaled or even absorbed through the skin but swallowing is the most common. Accidental poisoning is most common in young children. It is important to keep medications, cleaning agents and organic solvents out of a child's reach. If poisoning occurs, do not panic. Find out, if you can, what poison has been swallowed. Contact your doctor or the poisons information people immediately. Remember it is important to tell them which substance has been swallowed. Take the container, with any leftover substance, with you to the hospital. Sometimes a specific antidote may be available.

You may be told to induce vomiting if the substance does not contain any acid, alkali or petroleum product. However, this must be definitely confirmed as vomiting these substances will cause damage to the lungs and food pipe. Milk may help to neutralise the effects of corrosive substances. Give nothing by mouth for poisoning by petroleum-based products.

Drowning is a very common, and largely preventable, cause of death in young children. This is one accident that is clearly best dealt with by preventive measures such as adequate supervision, fencing of swimming pools and ensuring that children learn to swim as early as possible

Choking

The first sign that someone is choking might be a coughing fit, alarming attempts to breathe, clutching at the throat and increasing blue colour of the lips, face and nail beds. Try to get the person to relax, breathe deeply and cough up the obstruction. If this is not successful, three or four sharp blows between the shoulder blades may help. If the victim is breathing and unconscious, place him in the recovery position, on his side, and seek medical help.

COMMONLY PRESCRIBED DRUGS

Your doctor will explain: ❑ how the medication does its job ❑ common side effects that could develop ❑ how often to take the medication and its relation to meals ❑ any interactions with other medications ❑ when to come and see the doctor again

Antibiotics

There is a great variety of antibiotics available to treat bacterial infections. Viral infections are not helped by antibiotics. If your child presents to the doctor with what looks like an infection, uppermost in your doctor's mind will be whether the infection is likely to be caused by bacteria or a virus. If the doctor decides the infection is bacterial, antibiotics will be prescribed, if viral they will not. The site of an infection gives clues as to the most likely organism responsible for the infection.

Different organisms respond to different antibiotics and this will determine the particular antibiotic prescribed. Sometimes a sample may be taken from the infected area and sent to the laboratory for analysis. Even then, it is usual to begin treatment with antibiotics before the results are known, as this usually takes a few days. The choice of antibiotic will be based on the doctor's experience of the most likely infecting organism. Tetracyclines should not be given to children.

Antihypertensives

This is the name given to the large and diverse collection of drugs prescribed to lower blood pressure. It is customary to start with one drug and add others in a stepwise fashion or change to a new drug if blood pressure control is not satisfactory. Prescribing for blood pressure is an individualised process. Factors such as age, severity of the hypertension, other conditions suffered by the patient and any other drugs being taken, need to be considered. Not all drugs are suitable for everybody, as each has a number of precautions associated with its use. For instance, the beta-blocker group of drugs should not be used by anyone who has had asthma.

Anti-inflammatory drugs

Drugs from this group are prescribed to alleviate joint inflammation in arthritis or inflammation associated with muscle, tendon or joint injury. New formulations are continually becoming available. The newer drugs in this group need to be taken less often than the older types. All of them can cause irritation of the stomach lining, so they should be taken on a full stomach. Generally, anyone with a peptic ulcer cannot take medications from this group, but if they are necessary, careful medical supervision is required. Additional medication may also be prescribed to protect the stomach or intestinal lining. Alternative forms of medication, such as suppositories and sprays, may be considered.

Anti-asthma drugs

Many of the anti-asthma drugs are now prescribed in inhalant form. This allows the active ingredient to quickly reach the areas where it is required. There are a number of different types of asthma sprays containing different ingredients. Sprays containing cortisone reduce inflammation. Disodium cromoglycate sprays act as a preventative and bronchodilators act to widen the narrowed airways. It is not unusual to be prescribed a mixture of these medications, which will interact to decrease asthma symptoms in slightly different ways.

Cortisone creams

Creams containing cortisone are often prescribed for skin problems. It is important to remember that even though they are in a cream form, they should be treated with proper respect. They come in differing strengths, and cannot be applied just anywhere. Only the milder strength cream should be applied to the face, and all creams should only be used for short periods of time, unless otherwise instructed. Use them only for the situation for which they were prescribed. If cortisone is applied to infected or fungal lesions the condition will worsen.

Minor tranquillisers

These are mainly prescribed to treat anxiety. Those most commonly prescribed are from the benzodiazepine group of drugs. In general, this group of drugs should only be used for short periods of time as dependence can develop and withdrawal from the drugs can involve symptoms of anxiety and sleeplessness. The same group of drugs is used in most commonly prescribed sleeping tablets. Again, take these drugs for short periods only and reduce the dose slowly under medical direction. It is most important that minor tranquillisers and sleeping tablets are not stopped suddenly. Many people confuse minor tranquillisers with major tranquillisers and antidepressant drugs. These two groups are chemically different and are used in slightly different ways. Ask your doctor if you do not know which of these drugs you are taking.

Oral contraceptives

These are prescribed not only for contraception but for many period problems, such as pain or heavy blood loss.

COMMON NONPRESCRIPTION DRUGS

These days many drugs are available without prescription from chemists, health food stores and even supermarkets. Some of these have a useful place in the treatment of pain and minor disorders. Others are at best, of little value and at worst, dangerous.

Antihistamines

These drugs are used to treat allergies and hay fever. There is a large number of these preparations on the market so consult your doctor if you are confused. Some of the newer formulations do not cause drowsiness, a side effect often associated with antihistamines in the past. If you are taking a medication that causes drowsiness, do not drive a car or operate any machinery.

Cough mixtures

The market is flooded with cough mixtures, many of dubious value. There are two types of cough and a different cough mixture is best suited to each. One cough is productive, in which the cough is trying to get rid of an inhaled foreign body or mucus; the other type is nonproductive and is dry and irritating. Expectorant cough mixtures aim to liquefy the mucus of a productive cough, making it easier to expel. Suppressants reduce the desire to cough in a nonproductive cough. For a productive cough, warm drinks and steam inhalations are helpful. Avoid smoke and smoking if you have a cough.

Antidiarrhoea medicines

Current medical thinking is that diarrhoea, especially in children, should not be treated with over-the-counter medication aimed at stopping the diarrhoea. Treat diarrhoea by diet, giving plenty of clear fluids and only dry biscuits, rice, toast and honey. Avoid fatty foods, dairy foods, fruit and vegetables. See your doctor if symptoms persist and your doctor may suggest using a special oral, rehydration solution, available from the chemist. Sometimes treatment is required but, more often than not, careful diet and preventing dehydration is all that is necessary.

Aspirin and paracetamol

These are probably the most commonly used nonprescription drugs. Aspirin and paracetamol can both be used to relieve minor pain and fevers. It is best not to give aspirin to children but to use paracetamol instead.

Vitamins and the placebo effect

There are an enormous number of vitamins available on the market and their sales involve a major industry. Many users of vitamins swear to their efficacy. However, to put it bluntly, extra vitamins taken, in other than deficiency diseases, end up in the sewer. However, many people feel better when they are taking vitamins – in fact, in some studies, giving a 'dummy pill' or placebo (a pill that doesn't contain medicine) is as effective as giving a drug. Don't underestimate the placebo effect of 'popping a pill'. Studies have proved that a placebo can give a great psychological lift. Your belief that the pill, the healer or the behaviour is working (known medically as a placebo response), is a very powerful aid to getting better. This would explain a large number of success stories reported in both medical and alternative health practices. So as a placebo, low dose vitamin intake may in fact do you some good. However, do not go overboard with too many vitamins, or too high a dose. Medical problems do arise with vitamin overdosage.

'Natural' remedies

The use of the word 'natural' has tremendous appeal to many people. When placed in front of food or tablets the product's saleability is enhanced. Many people will swallow 'natural' foods or tablets without bothering to find out what the ingredients really are. In reality, natural healing is providing the optimum environment for healing to take place. This means avoiding smoking, alcohol and stress, eating a healthy balanced diet, and getting adequate sleep and relaxation. Before you use any of these so-called 'natural products', give some thought as to why you might need it, if you do at all.

Herbs

Take care with herbal remedies. They are not tested to the same high standard as pharmaceuticals. A number of herbal remedies are known to be toxic, especially over a long period of time, as they accumulate in your body. In addition to the naturally occurring poisons present in some herbs, contamination from other ingredients may also occur. Children and babies should never be given herbal remedies.

Seasickness medication

This type of medication is available in an oral form and, more recently, in the form of a skin patch. This latter is generally attached behind the ear and releases its active ingredient through the skin. Take care using these medications. They can be harmful to anyone suffering an intercurrent illness, taking certain other medications or because of their age. Read the instructions on the packaging very carefully and check with your doctor if you have any doubt as to whether to use it.

Taking your medicine

It would seem to go without saying that prescribed medicines should be taken just as prescribed. However, studies have shown great differences in how people actually take their medicines when compared with how they have been told to take them. Some medicines, for example antibiotics, require the full course to be taken, irrespective of when the symptoms cease. Some medications need to be taken long term and others for only as long as the symptoms require. Always follow your doctor's advice and write down any instructions to help you to remember. Go back to your doctor if you are not clear about the instructions you have been given or if you have any unanswered questions.

When it comes to taking medicine, always follow your doctor's advice

Here are some simple rules to follow:

- You should always consult your doctor if you develop a new symptom, feel sick or develop a rash. It is important to do this rather than altering your medication, perhaps inappropriately. Your doctor may revise the diagnosis or treatment, based on this new information.
- Don't share medication with anyone else. You may have similar symptoms but a different ailment. Each person is prone to different side effects and interactions, especially if they are using other medications at the same time.
- Ask questions if you don't understand anything about your condition or your treatment. Write them down before you visit your doctor so you don't forget anything. It is difficult to take in everything at once, particularly under stress, so it's a good idea to have a friend or relative with you who can listen and help you to remember afterwards.
- Tell your doctor about any drug allergies or any previous problems you have had when taking medication. Remember to tell your doctor your whole medical history and any relevant family history as well.
- Tell your doctor if you may be pregnant or if you are breastfeeding. Even if there is a remote chance of pregnancy, your doctor must know. There are many drugs harmful to the unborn child, especially in the early stages. Nursing mothers should avoid certain drugs, since these will be passed to the baby through breastfeeding.
- Familiarise yourself with your own drug treatment. Know the names of your medications, why you are taking them and their side effects.
- If you're not happy with your doctor, seek out an alternative. There are plenty of doctors around, so look for one that suits you.

Safety first

- Keep all drugs in a safety cupboard, out of reach of children.
- Dispose safely of unused medication.
- Don't share medication.
- Don't take pills from an unlabelled container.
- If starting a new medication, check with your doctor or pharmacist as to whether it will affect your ability to drive, operate machinery or drink alcohol.
- Keep medications in a cool, dry place, not in the bathroom cabinet, which tends to be warm and humid.

Keep medication in a cool dry place, not in the bathroom cabinet which tends to be warm and quite damp

Sound sense with medications

- Medications should be respected. They are potentially powerful and when used incorrectly can cause harm.
- All medications taken in excess can cause toxic reactions. Ask for more information rather than risk making a mistake.
- Do not assume that medications you can buy without prescription are harmless. They can be harmful and can also interact in harmful ways with prescribed medications. Tell your doctor about any over-the-counter preparations you may be taking. For example, nonprescription medications for coughs, colds and seasickness can worsen glaucoma and endanger eyesight.
- Don't assume that anything is innocuous. Take the time to read the instruction leaflets that are often included with medications. If this raises any questions or doubts in your mind, ask your doctor to answer them.

You should always have a basic first aid kit in the house, ready to use in an emergency, and be well versed in first aid techniques. Every adult in your house should know how to perform mouth-to-mouth resuscitation.

FIRST AID

Resuscitation

The primary aim of resuscitation is to ensure that the patient gets adequate air into the lungs. Brain damage can follow a relatively short period without oxygen, so quick action is essential.

If the person is not breathing:

1 Check that there is no obstruction of the airway, such as false teeth, vomit or a foreign body. Make sure that the tongue is not causing an obstruction.
2 Lay the patient flat on the ground with the head tilted slightly backwards.
3 In the case of infants and small children, place your open mouth over the child's nose and mouth and gently huff air from your lungs into the child. Do this for about two seconds for each breath. You can check that the air is reaching the child's lungs by watching the rise and fall of the child's chest. Repeat this four or five times, then check to see if the child is breathing spontaneously. If not, keep going until it does.
4 For older children, place your mouth over their mouth only and pinch the nose to make sure that air does not escape through the nose. Follow the procedure described above for about three seconds for each breath.

If there is no pulse:

1 You can sometimes restart the heart with a firm thump to the lower front of the chest with the edge of your hand. If this is not successful, begin external cardiac compression immediately.
2 In young children, place your index and middle finger at the mid-point of the breastbone and push downwards quickly five times every three seconds. You should be moving the chest between one and two centimetres. Stop after five compressions to check if spontaneous breathing is present. If not, give three artificial breaths. Continue this procedure until medical help arrives or the patient breathes alone.
3 In older children, compress the chest with the heel of your hand about five times every four seconds. Continue the procedure as described for younger children, until the patient is breathing spontaneously or medical help arrives.

✚ YOUR FIRST AID KIT ✚

- ❑ Syrup of Ipecac to induce vomiting. Check with the poisons information service before inducing vomiting
- ❑ An antiseptic liquid and cotton wool balls
- ❑ A pair of square-ended tweezers, small enough to remove fine splinters
- ❑ A pair of scissors, for cutting bandages and removing clothes from a burn
- ❑ A selection of bandages, sticking plasters and lint
- ❑ A hot/cold pack for strains and sprains
- ❑ Pins for securing bandages and a strong cotton square for a sling
- ❑ A small pack of alcohol swabs, to quickly sterilise a needle or thermometer
- ❑ A thermometer and a medicine measure
- ❑ Infants and children's liquid paracetamol
- ❑ A treatment for rashes, stings and itches, such as calamine lotion
- ❑ A cooling anti-inflammatory preparation
- ❑ A syringe, without the needle, for administering medication quickly

YOUR BODY

It's an old saying, but true – 'look after your body and it will look after you'. In this chapter you will find out all about skin problems, ear and eye diseases, back problems and how to treat them. Plastic surgery offers you a chance to change parts of your body that you are not comfortable with.

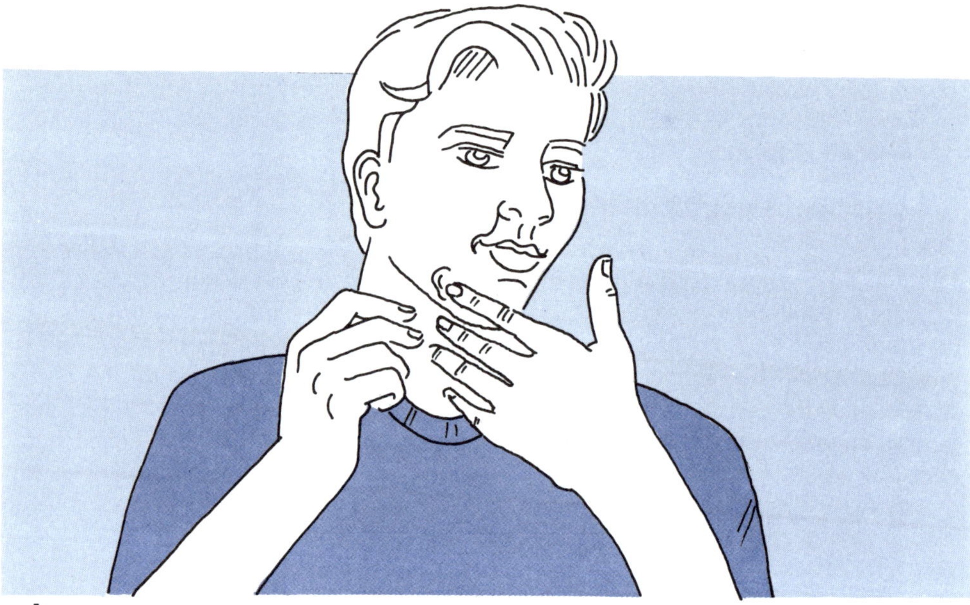

Skin

Acne

This common problem is often seen as the bane of adolescence. However, it can occur at any age, from shortly after birth to middle age. Acne, in the medical sense, covers the occasional pimple through to blackheads, whiteheads, cysts and swellings.

Acne is caused by a blockage in the opening of the oil glands on the skin. The tendency for this to occur is inherited. Blackheads are visible blockages that have become darkly pigmented. In whiteheads, the blockage is not visible but the small collection of oil under the skin is seen as a small white lump.

Inflamed red areas, often painful, are due to a rupture of the blocked gland under the skin. Pus may also be present. If the blockage occurs slightly deeper, then quite large cysts, which appear as red or pale lumps, can develop.

The most common place for acne to occur is on the face. It can also spread to the shoulders, back and chest. For those with susceptible skin, working in an oily environment may contribute to acne.

Treatment The usual way of managing acne is in a step-wise manner, proceeding from the simpler methods of control to the more complicated.

Firstly, if you must use cosmetics, avoid the oily ones in favour of water-based ones. There are a number of simple treatments, containing benzoyl peroxide or retinoic acid, that will solve the problem for many acne patients. It is important to observe instructions on use. Mild degreasing agents may also help. Soaps and solutions containing salicylic acid can improve the appearance, causing a mild peeling of the skin.

Certain antibiotics are also helpful. These are given in a lower dose than would be prescribed for an infection. Certain bacteria do find acne skin a pleasant environment. Their presence adds to the degree of inflammation present in acne. Hence, the eradication of these bacteria by antibiotics can help to settle the acne. The use of antibiotics probably reinforces the incorrect and cruel idea that acne is infectious and can be passed on to others. This is not the case.

Other treatments are available for severe acne that does not respond to any of the above treatments. The most recent development in this area is an oral medication called isotretinoin, derived from vitamin A. It has led many people to believe that vitamins may influence the course of acne. This is not so. The use of isotretinoin requires careful supervision. It must not be used during pregnancy as it can harm an unborn baby. It is absolutely essential that conception does not take place during the three or four months course of treatment and for some time after. This effect has restricted its use and at present isotretinoin can only be prescribed by a dermatologist. Chemical peeling and laser therapy may be helpful in some cases of intractable acne. Your doctor will be able to refer you to an appropriate specialist for these procedures.

Dermatitis and eczema

Dermatitis is an inflammation of the skin. Eczema is characterised by redness, swelling, oozing and blister formation. Laymen often use these terms interchangeably. There are many different types of dermatitis and only the more common are discussed here.

❑ ***Seborrhoeic dermatitis*** This form of dermatitis, characterised by scaling and inflammation of the scalp, face and occasionally other areas of the body, occurs in some people with oily skin. The mainstay of treatment is with cortisone-based creams. Treat scaly scalps with an anti-dandruff type shampoo.

❑ ***Contact dermatitis*** Many substances, such as soap solutions, shampoos, building materials, plants, jewellery and glues will cause skin irritation. If the substance can be identified and avoided, the problem can be solved. Cortisone creams are used to get inflammation under control. Oral antihistamines can reduce itching. In more severe cases, cortisone tablets may also be prescribed.

❑ ***Neurodermatitis*** Constant scratching can set up an area of 'neurodermatitis'. This is very often associated with, and a consequence of, emotional upset. Some areas of the body are more likely to be scratched than others, for example the neck, anus, vagina and scrotum.

❑ ***Eczema*** This is a very common condition that has a tendency to run in families and may be linked to a family or personal history of hayfever or asthma. Children may develop childhood eczema at a very early age. Eczema is not infectious nor is it a sign of lack of hygiene or neglect. The sufferer usually has dry skin that is fairly easily irritated and damaged. Avoid rough clothing, soap, chemicals and overheating. Bathing the affected area can be a problem. Check with your doctor as to how often and for how long you should bathe. It is important to keep your child from scratching the affected area. While there is no cure, eczema can be controlled by meticulous skin care and cortisone cream. Differing strengths of cortisone cream are prescribed for different parts of the body. Carefully follow your doctor's prescription when using these creams.

HELPING YOUR CHILD'S ECZEMA

❑ Control scratching
❑ Do not bathe too much or for too long
❑ Choose cotton or cotton mix clothing
❑ Avoid rough fabrics
❑ Be aware of stress
❑ Consult your doctor regularly and follow the treatment schedule suggested

ACNE: FACTS NOT MYTHS

❑ **Acne is contagious.** This is not true

❑ **Diet causes acne.** Many foods have been blamed for acne including chocolates, dairy foods, citrus fruits and cola. Diet does not influence most acne with the proviso that, if you notice a particular food worsens your acne, then by all means avoid it. As acne affects mainly adolescents, the emphasis on a healthy diet helps teenagers establish good eating habits. However, unnecessarily strict restrictions, that emphasise the feeling of being different from one's peers, are not helpful

❑ **Acne is caused by lack of cleanliness.** Acne is not related to dirt or grime on the skin's surface and in fact overzealous cleaning can make it worse

❑ **Sunlight is beneficial in the treatment of acne.** This is no longer believed to be the case. In fact, the medical profession is more concerned with the over-exposure to sunlight, risking skin cancer and premature ageing. In addition, with some of the medications used to treat acne, sunlight-induced rashes can be a side effect

❑ **Acne is caused by hormonal imbalance.** Acne is influenced by hormones but is not primarily a hormonal problem

MOLES AND CANCER

Increasing attention is being focused on skin cancer. Moles are quite common. Some can be present at birth while others develop later in life. Most are trivial but a very small percentage can become malignant or a new malignant mole can develop. If you notice any change in size or colour in an existing mole or notice a new, unusual mole, check with your doctor

Moles and blemishes

Moles Generally it is best to leave moles alone. However, if a change takes place in an existing mole, that is it darkens, bleeds, grows or becomes itchy, then you need immediate medical assessment. A new, rapidly growing mole or one that changes in colour and consistency also needs checking.

Blemishes There are a number of types of common skin blemishes.

❑ The port wine stain is a pigmented area present since birth. This disfiguring lesion, which does not disappear by itself, may be helped by laser therapy. Ask your doctor.

❑ Another commonly occurring blemish which appears a few weeks after birth is called a strawberry mark. This one does usually disappear of its own accord.

❑ Capillary telangiectasia are the fine red lines (capillaries) often found on the cheeks and nose.

❑ Spider naevi are small red areas with fine red lines radiating from the centre in a spider-like pattern.

❑ Some smaller leg veins closer to the surface are quite common and can be treated with injections.

❑ Certain birthmarks.

Laser treatment The types of skin blemishes best dealt with by laser therapy are those associated with excessive pigmentation or abnormally enlarged blood vessels, such as some of those listed above.

The treatment may require local anaesthesia or may not, depending on the site and the patient. The pain has been described as hot pins and needles. Many people, having heard of this treatment, regard it as the panacea for all skin ailments. The truth is its use is very restricted. If you believe you might benefit from this treatment, discuss the possibility with your doctor, who can then refer you if it is appropriate.

Sun care

It is imperative that everyone becomes aware of the need to protect themselves from the harmful effects of sunlight. No longer can those with more darkly pigmented skin that tans easily consider themselves safe. Skin cancer, related to sun exposure, is on the increase. With all the information available about premature ageing and skin cancer, the number of people who continue to worship the sun is amazing.

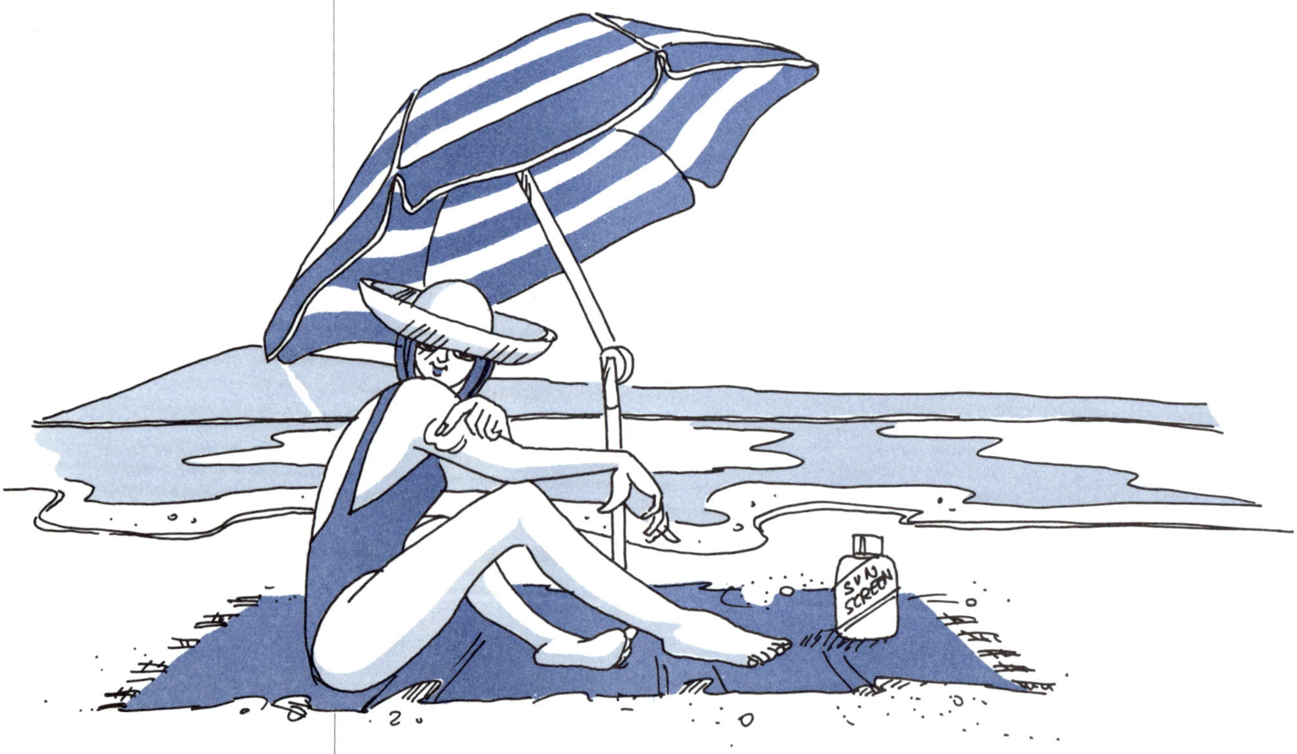

Plastic or cosmetic surgery

Cosmetic surgery tries to alter the person's appearance closer to the patient's ideal. Before undergoing cosmetic surgery, it is important that the prospective patient has a realistic understanding of what can be achieved. Cosmetic surgery will not make you beautiful if you are not beautiful to begin with. Like all surgery, it can be painful and complications can occur. The success of the surgery depends in part on the skill of the surgeon, but your own psychological make-up can also play a part. If you feel that the surgery makes you look better, then regardless of any objective assessment you are sure to feel better about yourself. In addition, it is expensive. The following are commonly performed procedures:

'Nose job' or rhinoplasty

This is the most popular cosmetic procedure. Plastic surgeons tend not to remove as much tissue and bone from the nose as they did earlier. The aim is now to produce a more natural-looking nose. Before the operation, you should discuss with the surgeon the shape of nose you want and whether it will suit your face. Sometimes the chin needs to be made more prominent (chin augmentation). Often a complaint of an apparently big nose may in fact be due to a receding chin. Techniques for chin augmentation surgery include silicone or bone implants as well as actually cutting in to the jaw bone and bringing it forward.

Body contouring or sculpting

This is the use of plastic surgery to reshape many different parts of the body. Many people wrongly see this as an easy alternative to losing weight. To achieve a good result you need to have lost the weight and have areas of overhanging skin. Scarring can be very bad if just fat is removed in obese people who don't have overhanging skin. The main areas treated with this type of surgery are:

- ***Arms*** Loose hanging skin can be tightened.
- ***Tummy tuck*** Weight loss or multiple pregnancies can result in unnecessary overhanging skin. Surgery involves a cut above the pubic area, beneath the bikini line. The umbilicus and excess skin are removed and the umbilicus repositioned. This is regarded as a major operation.
- ***Breast reduction*** Involves reshaping and repositioning the breast as well as removing tissue to make it smaller. The nipple can be repositioned so that nipple sensation and the ability to breastfeed can continue.
- ***Breast lifts*** Involve changing the position of the breast without changing its size.
- ***Breast enlargement*** Involves inserting a prosthesis into the breast to make it larger. Developments in this area have resulted in a softer, more natural breast.
- ***Breast reconstruction*** A great benefit to women who need removal of a breast (mastectomy). Surgery is often also needed to make the other breast equal in size and position in relation to the new breast.
- ***Suction lipectomy*** This a specialised technique for removing fat deposits. A small cut is made and a special cannula inserted through the cut. The amount of tissue removed can be as little as 30 to 40 g around the ankles to 3 or 4 kg from the abdomen. This technique does not correct loose skin but is most useful for the young who are not fat, have firm skin and a localised area of fat that they would like to get rid of. The areas of the body that are most suitable for this type of surgery are a double chin, in front of the arm pits, the lower stomach, hips and thighs. This treatment is not an alternative for weight loss. There are side-effects and complications, including local bruising, pain, swelling and skin irregularity in the early postoperative phase. It may take some weeks for the bruising to clear and some months for the skin irregularities to settle. Serious complications include infection and even death of underlying tissue.

FINDING YOUR SURGEON

- Ask around amongst your friends to learn from their experiences
- You will need a referral from your GP
- You can ask for a specific surgeon or be guided by your GP
- Shop around until you find a surgeon with whom you feel comfortable and confident

Face-lift

Also called rhytidectomy, this technique raises the facial skin to remove folds and lines. Neck, cheek and jaw are most often involved but forehead and eyebrows can also be treated.

The location of the cut depends on which area requires most skin removal. For males requiring a face-lift, it is important not to interfere with normal beard patterns. A face-lift will not create beauty where it was not present before and will last about eight to ten years. Those with fine wrinkled skin will have shorter-lived effects. Swelling, bruising and stiffness are most likely to occur as well as complications including bruising and infections. One of the potentially most serious side effects (fortunately rare), is the inadvertent cutting of facial nerves, resulting in a crooked smile or expression.

Dermabrasions and chemical face peel

Mechanical dermabrasion involves an instrument that effectively sands off the outer layer of the skin. The skin heals tighter. Often the procedure is carried out together with a face-lift. Chemical peeling uses a mixture that effectively burns off the outer layer of skin in a controlled way. It, too, heals with the skin appearing tighter. Again it is useful in conjunction with a face-lift. Olive and dark skin does not respond well to this form of treatment and a blotchy appearance may result.

Eye and eyebrow lift

Eye lift (or blepharoplasty) is one of the most successful plastic surgery procedures. The shape of the eyes will not change, but the eyes will look more youthful. Side effects include tearing or dry eyes and if the lower lid is pulled down too much, the whites of the eyes will be too obvious.

Raising the eyebrows can produce a more youthful and livelier appearance. Frown lines between the brows and across the forehead can also be removed. Unwanted complications include bruising, swelling and scars.

Ear correction

Otoplasty is a very successful operation that involves moving prominent ears closer to the head. Since the ear is fully grown by the age of six this procedure can save young people a lot of teasing.

Ears and eyes

Ear wax is a normal secretion, whose job it is to transport trapped dust and dirt particles to the outside. For most of us, this causes no problem. However, some people find that the wax dries on its way and blocks the canal, causing sudden deafness or blockage. It is wrong to self-medicate without the benefit of actually seeing what is happening in the ear; you should go to your doctor.

If the wax looks as if it needs softening, your doctor may suggest commercial ear drops or oil drops. The next step is to syringe the ear out, using water heated to body temperature. Sometimes this procedure needs to be repeated a few times.

Don't clean inside your ears. Nothing smaller than an elbow, in other words, nothing at all should enter the ear, since it has its own self-cleaning mechanism. Only the outer shell of the ear needs cleaning, with a damp cloth. Do not probe with cotton buds and matchsticks because you could push wax back into the ear or even pierce your eardrum.

Small children are the main culprits when it comes to pushing a variety of small objects into their ears. Syringing is often not advisable, particularly if the inserted material is vegetable matter, because it may swell, causing further complications. This is also true for insects that enter the ear. Don't try to deal with the problem by yourself; seek the help of a trained person

Middle ear infections

These are common in children aged less than ten years. So if you seem to be forever taking your child to the doctor for middle ear infections, take heart, as most of them do grow out of it. Infections are frequent because the passageways between ear, nose and throat are not fully developed in children and lie closer together. So nose and throat infections can easily make their way to the ear. Treatment will usually require an antibiotic for the infection and paracetamol for pain relief. Often a decongestant antihistamine is also given. It is important for the doctor to follow recurrent middle ear infections.

Glue ears

This develops when a thick, sticky, uninfected fluid collects behind the eardrum. There are no symptoms, but deafness is eventually noticed. The cause is not completely understood, but seems to relate to problems in the functioning of the Eustachian tube. Recurrent infection may also play a part. Repeated attacks of middle ear infections, together with Eustachian tube problems, prevent proper ventilation of the ear and could lead to long-term deafness. Treatment varies. Sometimes long-term medication is prescribed but often surgery to insert grommets (ventilation tubes) is required. The grommets generally fall out and the hole closes naturally.

Swimmer's ear

This is a different type of infection, involving the outer ear canal, which affects not only swimmers. The external canal of the ear becomes inflamed as a result of either bacterial, fungal, viral or chemical causes, resulting in itching, pain and discharge. Certain types of eczema can also cause the condition. Treatment involves the use of antibiotic drops as well as the removal of any excess material and discharge from the canal. Recurrent sufferers use special ear drops and insert plugs before swimming.

CLEANING EARS

Never insert cotton buds, matchsticks, hair pins or any other objects into the ear. A moist wash cloth to clean the outer shell is all that is necessary

COMMON EYE PROBLEMS

Problem	Characteristics	Treatment
Squint (lazy eye, strabismus, cast, turn or cross-eye)	Brain receives two images, but ignores image from the squinting eye. This can result in blindness in the eye	Corrected by glasses or a patch. Operation to straighten muscles that move the eye
Shortsightedness (Myopia)	Eyeball too long. Rare before school age, increasing to a peak at eleven years of age	Corrected by glasses. A new type of operation for adults whose short-sightedness falls within strictly defined criteria is now available
Longsightedness (hypermetropia)	Eyeball too short	Corrected by glasses
Astigmatism	The cornea varies in curvature. It can occur with long or shortsightedness	Corrected by glasses
Chronic simple glaucoma	Develops slowly without any signs and can result in loss of vision. Caused by slow rise in eye pressure for reasons unknown. Take care with over the counter preparations, such as cough medicine	Detected by frequent checks with specialist eye doctor (Ophthalmologist) every two years especially if forty years of age or over. Treated with eyedrops and oral medication
Cataracts	A cloudiness or thickening in the lens of the eye. Can occur through accident or develop with advancing age or be present from birth	Removal, if interfering with vision, and replacement with glasses, contact lens or a plastic lens implant. Risk of surgery will be balanced against better vision before deciding to operate
Diabetic eye disease	A condition in which blood sugar can affect the eyes – the longer diabetes lasts, the more the effect	Diagnosed by expert and regular check of eyesight. Treatment is by physical methods, such as laser

Back problems

These days back problems are a major health issue for the patient who is suffering and for the community facing the costs of dealing with the problem. Back pain interferes with every part of your life and can be very debilitating.

Learning to look after your back may do a great deal to prevent recurrent back pain. The muscles that support the spine and the abdominal muscles provide important support for the back. It is crucial that these muscles are exercised and strengthened.

When you visit your doctor, he or she will want to know if the back pain is associated with any other problems such as abdominal pain, nausea, vomiting, diarrhoea, bladder problems, flu symptoms, menstrual problems or whether you have had a recent injury or done unusual work.

Treatment For back pain due to muscle strain, treatment is conservative and includes the following:

- Resting flat on your back to relieve the muscle strain.
- Pain relief with a special heat lamp, hot water bottle and analgesics.
- Medications to reduce muscle tension.
- Anti-inflammatory drugs, including aspirin, ibuprofen, diflunisal and naproxen, may also be given. Different preparations will suit different people but some can cause nausea and vomiting. People who have had an ulcer, or gastrointestinal bleeding, are advised not to take these tablets. They always need to be taken on a full stomach to minimise the possibility of stomach irritation.
- Physiotherapy

Other treatments for chronic back pain are hospitalisation, traction and surgery.

LIFT RIGHT

- Assess the job – get help or a trolley if you need to
- Lift smoothly, don't jerk suddenly
- Bend your knees before you lift. Use your legs not your back
- Hold the weight close to your body for added support

BASIC BACK CARE

- Maintain good posture at all times. This keeps the spine in the best position, puts least strain on the discs and improves breathing and circulation
- Learn how to lift correctly. Always think about how you are going to lift before you do it. If the object is too heavy, ask for help
- Sit with your back straight in a chair which supports the lower back. Sit right back in the chair with your feet resting on the floor. If needed, support the curve of the lower back with a small cushion
- Use a firm mattress or a board under the mattress to provide back support. Don't lie on your stomach as this increases the strain on your back
- Use a low pillow
- Give yourself instant relief by lying on the floor with your knees bent

Scoliosis

This is a lateral, or sideways, curve of the spine that develops in early adolescence. It is more common in girls, affecting about ten per cent, and tends to run in families. The cause is unknown. In only a small number of cases is the condition severe enough to require treatment.

The signs of scoliosis include:

- Head leans to one side
- One shoulder higher
- Unequal gaps between body and arms
- One arm seems longer
- One hip sticks out more

Treatment Adequate early detection and, if necessary, treatment can eliminate risk of pain, heart and lung problems and deformity later in life. A spinal brace may be needed. More rarely, surgery is required.

Feet and legs

Athletes foot

This is a fungal infection, usually between the toes or under the arch of the foot. It is often picked up in public swimming pools and showers and is aggravated by moisture. Treatment is directed towards keeping feet dry and cool. Choose cotton socks and avoid washing your feet in hot water. Some over the counter remedies, such as foot powders and creams, may be helpful.

Callus

This is a thickened area of skin, often on the ball and heel of the foot. It may not be painful and is a normal response to the area being constantly rubbed by ill-fitting shoes.You can carefully remove some of the dead skin but do not rub too vigorously. Use a moisturiser regularly. When buying new shoes, pay as much attention to the comfort of your feet as to the latest fashion trend. If the callus is causing a problem, a chiropodist (podiatrist) can remove it for you.

Corns

These are small, painful, cone-shaped areas of thickened skin that usually form at pressure areas. Tight footwear can contribute to the problem. Treatment by a chiropodist (podiatrist) and the use of corn pads may help.

Bunion (halux valgus)

This is the commonest foot deformity where the big toe points to the side. Women are more likely to develop this condition which runs in families. The development of the condition can be accelerated if the foot is continually squashed into narrow, high-heeled shoes. Surgery is the final option but there is a long recovery period and some possible complications.

Plantar warts

These are really no different from warts found on other parts of the body. They are caused by a virus. Pain occurs if they are present on the weight-bearing parts of the foot. They can be removed by slowly burning off with chemical treatments, freezing and surgery. Plantar warts, like other warts, may eventually disappear by themselves as your body develops resistance to them.

Varicose and spider veins

Varicose veins are stretched, enlarged veins caused by blood pooling in the veins because the valves that control the blood flow are not working properly. Vein disorders can run in families. Spending long periods of time on your feet will aid their development.

Spider veins are small purple veins in clusters just under the skin. These usually cause no symptoms but people find them unsightly and want to be rid of them.

Treatment Exercises that reverse the blood flow in the veins are helpful. Try lying on your back and resting your legs against a wall for a few minutes a couple of times a day. Support hose and bandaging is also helpful. If further treatment is required, then surgery to completely remove the veins is the usual method.

Spider veins can often be treated with an injection of a chemical substance that irritates the vein, causing it to disappear.

Conditions which affect varicose veins:

- prolonged standing
- pregnancy
- obesity
- inactivity
- thrombophlebitis

BASIC FOOT CARE

- Keep the skin soft and supple with a moisturiser
- Carefully wash and dry between the toes. Use methylated spirits between the toes
- Choose shoes with a good airflow and which allow movement of the toes

From the moment of birth, parents are concerned about their baby's health and development. Childhood seems to be a time of frequent, minor illnesses. It is also a period during which immunity to many common diseases develops.

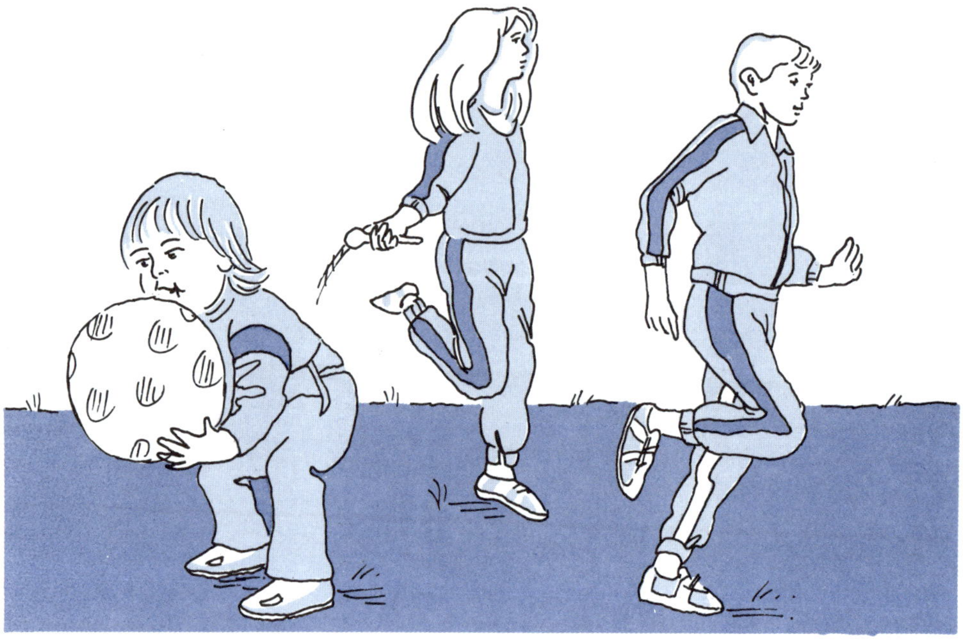

Your baby

Is my baby normal? This is the prime concern of all new parents, but bear in mind that babies and their development are very variable. If you are worried about your baby, you should seek answers. Your first call could be either the local Child Health Centre or your doctor.

Many parents are loathe to call the doctor 'unnecessarily'. Most parents show great common sense and do as much as they can to help their sick children. They should never hold off getting medical help for their child, or for that matter, for themselves. If you are worried and need reassurance, or another opinion, then you should have it. Some people feel they have been a nuisance if the doctor happens to agree with their diagnosis, but when you are carrying the responsibility of looking after a sick child, that reassurance is essential.

Most male babies are circumcised when only a few days old. It is probably much safer to perform the operation at about six months, when his immune system and clotting mechanisms have had a chance to mature

Circumcision

At present, most doctors are not in favour of routine circumcision on male infants, because they don't believe that there is any health benefit. Normal attention to cleanliness should keep the uncircumcised penis clean and free from infection in the majority of cases. Circumcision was introduced many years ago at a time when regular bathing was not common. Circumcision continues to be performed for cultural, ritual and religious reasons among some sections of the population. In addition, there are accepted medical reasons for performing circumcisions. These include a tight foreskin, which may make the passing of urine difficult, and repeated or severe infection.

Care of the uncircumcised penis does not require active pulling back of the foreskin for the first few years. After this time, the child should be shown how to pull the foreskin back gently to wash. Overly-vigorous activity can result in tears, in both senses of the word, and even difficulty in pulling back the foreskin as the boy gets older. Circumcision is not without risks. If the procedure is carried out, then it is safer after the newborn period.

Common infant problems

❑ ***Crying*** Although incessant or uncharacteristic crying can be a sign of illness, many healthy babies go through stages of crying. Parents are driven to the limits of their patience and trying to work out what is needed can be trial and error. Crying can be the baby's way of communicating a need for food, a clean nappy or comfort. Some babies need closer contact than others. One way of achieving this is to use a baby sling, which allows you to carry baby around and still get on with your work. You may find that wrapping baby securely can lessen its anxiety and stop the crying. Gentle noise is another trick that can be used to help baby settle and sleep. The radio, a tape of baby and mother's heartbeat, and even machine noise can be soothing. If boredom is a problem, break the baby's routine with a walk, or add some coloured toys and posters to liven up baby's scenery.

❑ ***Colic*** Colic has been around for a long time. The best thing that can be said about it is that it will pass. Although theories and treatments abound, it is not really known what causes colic. One theory (without substantiation) that has enjoyed popularity is that baby's digestive tract is causing the pain. Others contend that the baby is crying as a result of stress. Calm and reassurance is probably the best approach, stopping the vicious circle where parents become upset and accentuate the feelings of disquiet in the infant. While you are at it, reassure yourself that colic is not caused by bad parenting.

❑ ***Fever*** You should try to lower the temperature to prevent your child having a fever-related fit. Sponging or bathing your child with tepid water and giving paracetamol mixtures will help to bring fever down. Ensure that the child is having enough liquids – you don't have to worry about eating at this stage. Do not give compounds containing aspirin to children or adolescents, because a very rare but dangerous syndrome has been associated with aspirin usage in children.

❑ ***Diarrhoea and vomiting*** Again, make sure your child has an adequate intake of fluids to prevent dehydration in the acute stage. Eliminate dairy and fatty foods, most fresh fruit and vegetables. Check with your doctor about a suitable diet.

❑ ***Croup and coughing spasm*** Humidifying the air can help a lot. Turn on the hot water taps in the bathroom so that the room steams up, but take care to hold your child safely away from the hot water. Common colds and coughs can be treated with humidification while the child is sleeping, by buying or hiring a humidifier. If you are using steam inhalation to treat respiratory symptoms, make sure that you only use the sink, not a bowl full of hot water to produce steam. Accidents have occurred in which even teenagers and adults have been badly burnt by an overturned bowl of steaming water.

❑ ***Blocked nose*** Some doctors are not fans of nose drops. Overenthusiastic use can cause problems. However, babies who are unable to eat, drink or sleep because of a blocked nose, can be given a small dose of paediatric strength nose drops for short periods only. Try humidifying the air (as described above) first.

❑ ***Overweight babies*** Having a bit of extra weight can be handy if baby becomes sick, but it is wise not to allow your baby to become obese. Do not, under any circumstances, place a baby or child on a diet without first consulting your doctor.

PREVENTING OBESITY BEGINS IN BABYHOOD

❑ Establish good food patterns early in life

❑ If using formula, make sure that it is made up according to instructions

❑ Don't thicken bottle feeds with cereals, rusks and biscuits

❑ Don't feed babies or small children sugared foods such as cordials, soft drinks, lollies, sweet biscuits or cakes

❑ Don't give your child fried fatty foods such as chips and pastries

❑ Teach your child to eat fresh fruit rather than to drink highly sweetened fruit juices

COPING WITH A CRYING BABY

Once you are sure your baby is not hungry or needs changing, try:

❑ Swaddling the baby securely in a blanket

❑ Soft music, low continuous machine noise or 'heart beat' tapes

❑ De-stress the environment (including yourself) as much as possible

❑ Carrying baby in a sling or an outing in the pram or the car

Do not, under any circumstances, place a baby or child on a diet without first consulting your doctor

Childhood infections

❑ ***Chicken pox*** This is a common, acute, very infectious, viral disease – also called varicella zoster. It usually occurs between two and eight years. The symptoms include fever, a feeling of being unwell and an itchy rash. Fortunately, complications do not often occur. There is no specific treatment. Paracetamol may be given for fever and discomfort, antihistamines and lotions may be suggested for the itch. The child is no longer contagious once the skin lesions have dried. This usually takes between five and ten days from the first signs of the rash.

❑ ***Rubella or German measles*** This common infection is important because of the disastrous effects it can have on unborn babies if a pregnant woman becomes infected. It is normally a fairly mild illness. Many people aren't even aware that they have had it. Others develop noticeable symptoms – fever, swollen lymph glands and a rash.

Treatment is aimed at decreasing the discomfort of symptoms. The disease is no longer infectious after the fifth day. Rubella is important as a public health issue. The current aim is to vaccinate all children. A booster is required in early adolescence.

❑ ***Measles*** Measles is a widespread infectious disease. It is usual for babies to be immunised against measles. Young infants are protected to some degree by antibodies from their mother even before vaccination. Most cases of measles are straightforward but serious complications can occur. Symptoms include fever, cough, cold symptoms, sore eyes and a rash. Give paracetamol to decrease fever and discomfort. Measles is no longer infectious five days after the rash appears.

❑ ***Mumps*** Mumps is usually an infection of the salivary glands. It is often a mild disease, but there is a danger to adolescent and adult males if the testicles become infected, resulting in sterility. Many people can have the illness without knowing it. Headache, fever and painful swelling of the salivary glands are the most common symptoms. Treatment is to ease the discomfort of the sufferer with adequate pain and fever relief, coupled with rest and fluids. Children aged fifteen months are usually immunised against mumps together with the vaccine for measles and German measles.

❑ ***Roseola*** This is a common, benign, viral illness that causes fever and rash in children under two years. It can be confused with measles. Treatment to lower fever and discomfort is all that is required.

❑ ***Erythema Infectiosum*** Also known as 'slapped face syndrome' or fifth disease. The infected child can be recognised by the distinctive redness on the cheeks. It really does look as if someone has slapped his or her face. The rash spreads from the face and can last a couple of days. The illness is accompanied by fever, headache, loss of appetite and sore joints.

❑ ***Glandular fever*** A common disease caused by the Epstein-Barr virus (EBV), it occurs most commonly in adolescents and young adults. The virus, found in the salivary glands, is often passed on by close contact, such as kissing, but can also be transmitted by coughing. Symptoms include a feeling of being very tired, lacking energy, generalised pain, fever, swollen glands and a very sore throat. Complications can include respiratory obstruction if the throat is very swollen, liver and spleen involvement, and secondary bacterial throat infections. This can make the diagnosis and treatment rather difficult.

The treatment for glandular fever is basically adequate rest and fluids, and paracetamol for fever and pain. An antibiotic is not needed because the infection is caused by a virus. However, if a secondary bacterial infection develops, then antibiotics will be needed. Because the infection can either drag on for a long time or recur, it is important the sufferer should have adequate rest, avoid alcohol and have a healthy diet for a number of months after the illness, preferably for life.

❑ ***Acute gastroenteritis*** This infection occurs very commonly in children. Its onset can be sudden, with an otherwise well child developing vomiting, diarrhoea and fever. In severe cases, dehydration can develop quickly. The important thing is to prevent dehydration. Special oral rehydration powders are available. These replace

ANTIBIOTICS

Antibiotics are not helpful in a viral infection, only for those infections caused by bacteria. If your doctor does prescribe an antibiotic, it is essential to take the full course unless side effects develop. Never give your child antibiotics that have been prescribed for you

Traditionally, flat lemonade has been given to children as a treatment for diarrhoea or acute gastroenteritis. This is no longer thought to be safe. Instead, dilute one part lemonade in four parts water or give one teaspoon of sugar in one cup of water

the essential minerals and ingredients that can very quickly become lost with repeated vomiting and diarrhoea. Check with your doctor as to whether these powders are appropriate in your particular circumstances.

Although children may not feel like eating in the acute period, it is important that they take fluids. Your family doctor should be able to provide you with a suitable diet sheet. Generally, you should avoid all fatty and dairy foods, vegetables and fruit. Foods that can be eaten include toast, honey, jam, dry biscuits, rice, poached fish or chicken. It is not usual to prescribe medicines for acute gastroenteritis. Careful management of the diet, plenty of fluids and close observation are the mainstays of treatment. See your doctor if symptoms persist.

COMMON ILLNESSES OF CHILDHOOD

Chickenpox	No specific treatment – paracetamol can be given for fever and discomfort, and antihistamines and lotions for the itch
Rubella or German Measles	The discomfort of symptoms should be eased
Measles	Paracetamol can be given to decrease fever and discomfort
Mumps	Treatment to decrease fever and discomfort
Roseola	Treatment to decrease fever and discomfort
Erythema Infectiosum (slapped face syndrome)	Treatment to decrease fever and discomfort
Glandular Fever	Adequate rest. Fluids and paracetamol can be given for fever and pain
Acute Gastroenteritis	Dehydration should be prevented (oral rehydration powders mixed with water are recommended). Fatty and dairy foods, vegetables and fruit should be eliminated in the beginning

Note: This table includes only a summary of treatments. Consult your doctor if you are concerned

Vaccination

Routine immunisation has had a tremendous impact on the reduction of disease. Immunisation can have side effects and, very occasionally, these can be serious. However, the chances of contracting the disease and suffering serious complications are much higher than the chances of side effects from the vaccination. In some parts of the world, it is compulsory that each child presents documentary evidence of having been adequately immunised before starting school.

Unfortunately, there has been some irresponsible media reporting which has led directly to a fall in immunisation rates. In Britain, an epidemic of whooping cough, with associated deaths, has been linked to a fall in immunisation rates following a television documentary on the subject. This kind of unbalanced and irresponsible reporting is hazardous to our children's health by causing anxiety and confusion in parents. Having your child immunised is traumatic enough without being fed negative and unscientific information by the media.

Parents should make sure that the whole family is fully immunised. Discuss with your doctor what you have read or seen and any fears you may have. Once you fully understand the benefits of immunisation, you will have no difficulty in making your decision.

COUGHS AND COLDS

You may find that you seem to be constantly visiting the doctor with your young children during their frequent colds. Fortunately, most children will grow out of this unhappy tendency. It seems that the child's young immune system needs that time to develop resistance to the viruses common in the environment

IMMUNISATION IS ESSENTIAL

- It reduces the incidence of disease
- It reduces the length and severity of disease
- While there is a very small risk of serious side effects with whooping cough vaccine, the chances of suffering serious problems are much greater if an unvaccinated child catches whooping cough

Illnesses prevented by immunisation

- ***Diphtheria:*** The number of children dying from this disease has dropped dramatically since the introduction of the vaccine. Occasionally, mild side effects are associated with immunisation, including slight fever, headache and tiredness. Adults should receive booster vaccinations.
- ***Tetanus*** Vaccination against tetanus has been very successful in reducing the incidence of the disease which can occur after fairly mild wounds. The whole community should be immunised against tetanus.
- ***Whooping cough*** The death rate from this very serious disease is estimated to be 1:500 children under one year and 1:2500 children of all ages. The vaccination has a very low rate of serious side effects. If you catch the disease naturally, the chances of developing serious problems are higher than the chances of harmful side effects of vaccination. Very few children cannot be immunised. The vaccination is not totally protective. However, if a vaccinated child catches the disease, it is usually shorter and less severe than in an unvaccinated child.
- ***Polio*** Polio has virtually disappeared since the introduction of the oral vaccine. If you have not been vaccinated, or can't remember, be immunised with your child, as long as you are not pregnant.
- ***Measles vaccine*** Natural measles carries a risk of severe complications, but the risks of complications after the injection are much less. About six to nine days after

CHILDHOOD IMMUNISATION SCHEDULE

Age	Disease	Vaccine	Route of Administration
2 months	Diphtheria, tetanus, pertussis, Poliomyelitis	Triple antigen Sabin vaccine	Intramuscular Oral
4 months	Diphtheria, tetanus, pertussis, Poliomyelitis	Triple antigen Sabin vaccine	Intramuscular Oral
6 months	Diphtheria, tetanus, pertussis, Poliomyelitis	Triple antigen Sabin vaccine	Intramuscular Oral
12-15 mths	Measles/mumps/rubella	Measles/mumps/ rubella vaccine	Subcutaneous
18 months	Diphtheria, tetanus, pertussis	Triple antigen	Intramuscular
5 years (prior to school entry)	Diphtheria, tetanus, Poliomyelitis	Combined diph-theria and tetanus Sabin vaccine	Intramuscular Oral
10-15 years (females only)	Rubella	Rubella vaccine	Subcutaneous
15 years (or prior to school exit)	Diphtheria, tetanus	Adult diphtheria/ tetanus	Intramuscular

the injection, some children will develop fever and maybe a rash, lasting a few days. Other reactions are rare. The vaccine is usually given at twelve to fifteen months. The older the child the better the protection, but the child could develop the disease while waiting to be immunised.

❑ ***Mumps*** A study has shown that vaccination against this disease has resulted in a lower incidence of mumps-related meningitis.

❑ ***Rubella (German measles)*** This is a fairly mild disease but, if contracted by a pregnant woman, can cause serious defects in the unborn child. Teenage girls, and more recently babies, are now being vaccinated, further reducing the incidence of rubella-caused defects.

Immunisation of babies against measles, mumps and German measles may not last a lifetime. In the future, teenage boys and girls may be given a second dose.

❑ ***Hepatitis B*** Vaccination is available for those at high risk of developing the disease: health care workers; intravenous drug abusers; haemodialysis patients; homosexuals; those living with a carrier or someone in a high risk category and the sexually promiscuous. There is still argument as to whether the whole community should be vaccinated. Not everyone who is immunised will develop immunity. A booster may be necessary every three to five years after the initial three injections, to give continued protection.

❑ ***Haemophilus influenza type B*** In the US and Finland, three doses of vaccine are given during the first year of life to protect against this respiratory disease.

Allergies

In times past and before modern treatment became available, people would hang wet sheets across windows in order to trap the airborne particles that caused hayfever. It probably helped to reduce the problem somewhat but as we now know, allergy-causing particles do not only reach us through the air.

Tell your doctor about any allergies you may have, especially allergy to medications

Allergy is becoming an increasingly popular diagnosis, often made inappropriately by nonmedical people. In particular, both children and adults may then be placed on unnecessarily harsh diets or restrictions. Never place your child on a diet without first consulting your doctor.

The allergic response is really a series of chemical responses by your body to get rid of the offending agent or 'allergen'. Our bodies mount an attack against harmful substances like viruses, bacteria and tumour cells. But why some people's bodies also try energetically to get rid of harmless substances, such as grass, dust and strawberries, is not really known.

Remember to tell your doctor if you are allergic to any medication. Don't assume that they know. Taking medication to which you are allergic can be life threatening.

Symptoms of an allergic reaction

An allergic reaction can produce many different symptoms depending on which part of the body reacts. Originally it was noticed that during the 'haymaking' season people would develop symptoms of sneezing, itching and nasal stuffiness due to the presence of pollens in the air – hence hay fever.

Asthma, eczema and, more rarely, gastrointestinal symptoms can develop as part of an allergic response. There are many different types of allergens. Some are inhaled such as dust, animal hair, pollens and fungi, and some are ingested in medications or foods. The tendency to develop certain allergic diseases often runs in the family.

Hay fever sufferers may develop polyps (swellings in the linings of the nose) which can be removed surgically.

What are you allergic to?

By observing what brings on your allergic symptoms, you may be able to answer this question for yourself, or it may be necessary to undergo skin and blood tests. Food allergy is a difficult one to solve and you should have proper medical tests before making your own, or someone else's, life miserable with unnecessary food restrictions. Two techniques are used in assessing a true food allergy. One is a well-supervised elimination diet, that includes foods which are usually known not to cause food allergy and eliminating those foods that often are. The other, the Provocative Food Test, involves the introduction of foods one at a time to see if they do provoke the allergic reaction.

STEPS TO DETERMINE THE CAUSE OF YOUR ALLERGY

Be observant to the cause of your allergy, eg. medications, food, dust, animal hair, pollens. A medical investigation may be necessary involving

- ❑ skin and blood tests
- ❑ well-supervised medical elimination diet
- ❑ Provocative Food Test

Treatment As a first step, avoid whatever is causing the allergic reaction. This may or may not be possible. For example, avoiding dust is not easy. In addition, it is sometimes possible to be desensitised, either by injection or ingestion. This involves giving small amounts of the offending agent over a period of time to build up a tolerance to it. The injections seem to work best for people with seasonal grass pollen allergy. The desensitising injections should be given each year before the pollen season starts.

There are also a number of medications that can help. Here is a brief guide to allergy medications:

❑ ***Antihistamines*** These work quite well in preventing sneezing and running noses but can cause sleepiness. Finding one to suit you is a matter of trial and error, but the newer antihistamines are less likely to cause drowsiness.

❑ ***Decongestant nasal sprays*** Will help to clear a blocked nose but should only be used for short periods. If used for too long and then stopped, the nose becomes even more blocked.

❑ ***Preventative nasal sprays*** These contain similar drugs to those used in asthma sprays. Regular usage is needed for effect. In general, you require a doctor's prescription for these.

DEALING WITH ALLERGY

- ❑ Avoid the cause if possible
- ❑ Try desensitising injections if you can't avoid the cause
- ❑ Ask your doctor about appropriate medication

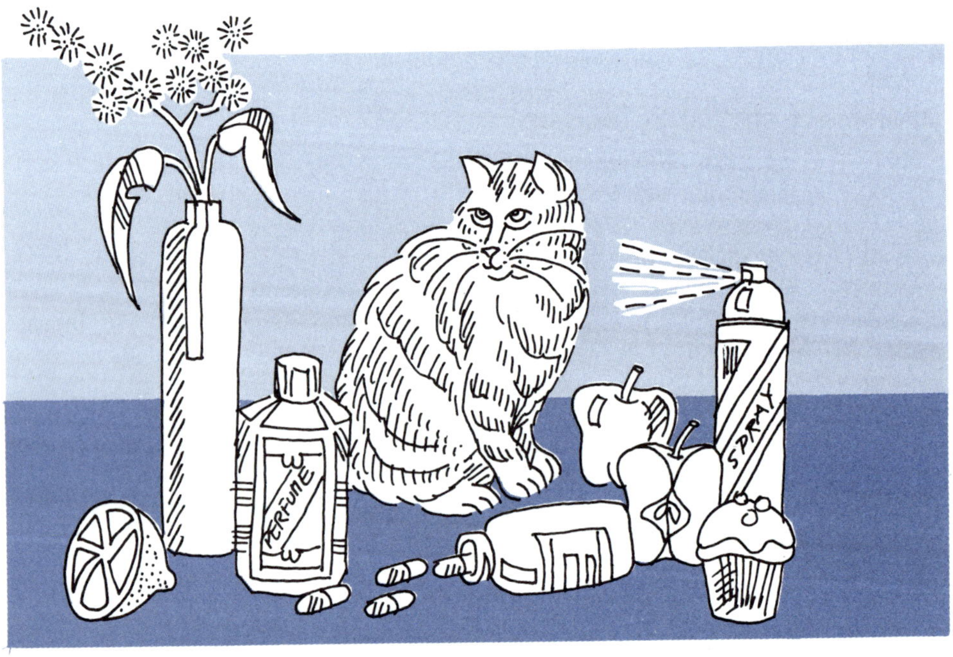

Asthma

Asthma should not be underrated – it is a potentially fatal condition. As many as 1:5 preschoolers suffer from asthma. Many infants will grow out of the condition. Doctors and parents alike have been loathe to use the term asthma for these little ones, preferring terms like allergic bronchitis, wheezy bronchitis or asthmatic bronchitis. Many young children only wheeze when they have an upper respiratory tract infection. These children have a very good chance of growing out of their asthma attacks later in childhood.

There are many things we still don't know about asthma. For example, no one knows why some cultural groups are more likely to suffer from asthma than others. It is also not possible at this stage of knowledge to predict who will outgrow the disease or who might die from it. It is even sometimes difficult to obtain accurate figures on incidence, because of the many labels applied to asthma.

What actually happens in asthma?

During an asthma attack the airways become narrower, so that breathing is difficult. The 'wheezing' sound is the noise caused when the air passes through the narrowed and swollen airway.

WHAT BRINGS ON AN ASTHMA ATTACK?

- exercise
- allergy (including inhaled substances, drugs and foods)
- infection
- weather changes
- stress

What to do in a crisis

You should always anticipate a crisis. Ask your doctor for a personal crisis plan and seek medical care as soon as possible. Teenagers appear to be at special risk because so often they ignore their disease, adopting a bravado attitude with dangerous results. Asthma is a chronic condition that should be taken seriously.

Exercise and asthma

You can prevent exercise-induced asthma by taking medication before starting the exercise. Warming-up before starting to exercise can also be helpful. Not all forms of exercise will induce asthma in those susceptible to it. Swimming is regarded as an excellent form of exercise for sufferers of asthma.

Managing your asthma

Even very small children can be taught to participate in the management of their illness. Obviously, the older the child, the more responsibility they can take.

There are many different types of medications which prevent or control the condition. Discuss a plan of management with your doctor. This may involve taking one or more drugs at the same time every day. It is vital that you use medications as directed, or you reduce their effectiveness and put yourself at risk. For more information on drugs to treat asthma, see Remedies, page 16.

You can buy yourself a peak flow meter. This is a simple tube attached to a machine into which you breathe. It can monitor the severity of an asthmatic attack by measuring the openness of the airways.

Make sure that you take your prescribed medications regularly.

Be familiar with your personal crisis plan. Any change in your asthma should be reported to your doctor.

Get in touch with an asthma group which, amongst other things, provides information, may organise children's holiday camps and may produce a journal.

WHAT TO DO

- Sit the patient down comfortably
- Offer reassurance
- Stay calm
- If the patient uses a bronchodilator, make sure it's available
- Use a peak flow meter to check progress
- Get medical help if symptoms do not subside

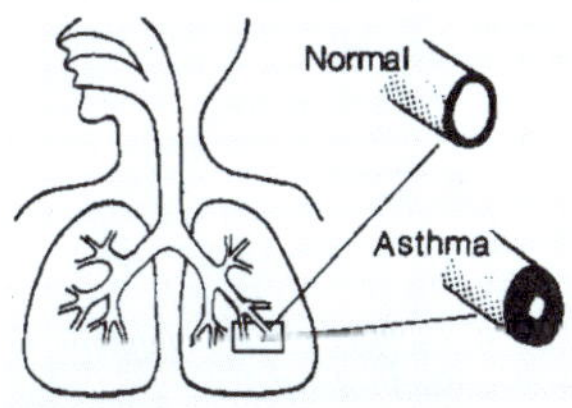

Illustration of lungs showing bronchial tubes as they appear normally and during an attack of asthma

Common childhood complaints

Warts

Most people are surprised to find that warts are a type of viral infection. Folklore abounds with picturesque remedies. Many people are impatient to be rid of these unsightly, but generally symptom-free, blemishes. There are some paints on the market which burn off the offending wart over a few months. It is important to be aware of their burning effect and to ensure that the normal skin surrounding the wart is protected. You can do this by sticking a small piece of plaster on the skin with a hole cut out for the wart to go through. Sometimes the treatment proposed for warts is worse than the condition. Burning or surgically removing them is no guarantee of a cure and may result in scarring. Left alone, your body will eventually develop an immunity to the virus, and your warts will disappear.

Molluscum contagiosum

This is another viral skin infection quite common in children under the age of five years. It often occurs as a crop of small pearly to pink raised lesions in the upper part of the body or the face. Take heart, they usually disappear without treatment. Your doctor can speed the process by piercing the lesions and painting them with iodine. This is a little painful and generally not worth the effort.

Growing pains

Many children, who are otherwise well, awaken periodically complaining of 'sore legs'. The pain responds to paracetamol, stroking and reassurance. If your doctor is satisfied that nothing else is wrong, he or she may diagnose 'growing pains'. Many experts say growth is not supposed to be painful but no alternative explanation is available. Be reassured, this recurrent distressing condition will eventually disappear.

Hyperactivity

The term 'hyperactivity' has been used indiscriminately in our community to describe a very difficult child. Families with other emotional problems have seized upon the idea that their child is hyperactive when it is often other members of the family, or family issues, that need attention.

Treatment Perhaps the most popular treatment has involved changing the diet. The Feingold diet which is free of additives and preservatives is very popular with the public but health care professionals are less enthusiastic about its claims. Diet management, as well as drugs, psychiatric and psychosocial modification, are all helpful in dealing with behavioural problems in children. If you believe that a child in your family is hyperactive, consult your doctor. Never manipulate a child's diet without medical supervision.

Puberty

There is a great range of what is normal development at puberty. The tables here are only a guide as to what to expect.

Lack of development If your daughter has not shown any changes of puberty by the time she is thirteen-and-a-half years old, or your son by the time he is fourteen years old, or if your child starts developing and then stops for a couple of years, it is time to see your doctor. In many cases, your child may be just developing slowly or maturation may be delayed due to some other factor, such as illness. Your doctor will want to do a blood test to check hormone levels.

It is worthwhile looking at your family history. Finding out that parents also took a long time to develop can reassure a child.

PROBLEMS OF PUBERTY

Puberty is more than a series of physical changes

- It is a time of testing independence
- New relationships are being tried, especially with the opposite sex
- Sometimes physical changes can cause embarrassment and uncertainty
- Teenagers often challenge authority at home and school

CLASSIFICATION OF GENITAL MATURITY STAGES IN BOYS

Age	Pubic Hair	Penis	Testes
0-8yrs	None	Preadolescent	
Approx 12yrs	Scanty, long slightly pigmented	Slight enlargement	Enlarged scrotum pink, texture altered
Approx 15yrs	Resembles adult type, but less in quantity, coarse, curly	Larger, glans and breadth increase in size	Larger, scrotum dark
Approx 18yrs	Adult distribution, spread to medial surface of thighs	Adult	Adult

CLASSIFICATION OF GENITAL MATURITY STAGES IN GIRLS

Age	Pubic Hair	Breasts
0-8yrs	None	Preadolescent
Approx 12yrs	Sparse, lightly pigmented, straight, medial border or labia	Breast and papilla elevated as small mound, areolar diameter increased
Approx 14yrs	Coarse, curly, abundant but amount less than in adult	Areola and papilla form secondary mound
Approx 17yrs	Adult feminine triangle, spread to medial surface of thighs	Mature, nipple projects, areola part of general breast contour

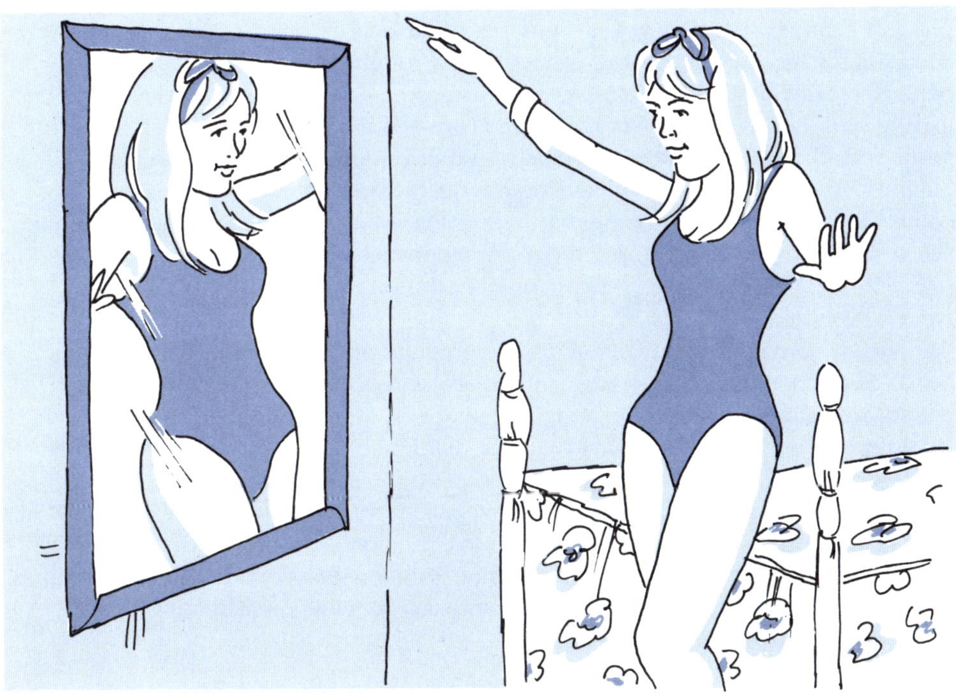

GENITAL MATURITY

Remember any timetable of maturational milestones is only a guide. There is a great range of what is normal. Discuss any worries with your doctor

These days women are being encouraged to be more open about health issues that concern them. Finding a doctor with whom you feel comfortable discussing personal matters is an important step.

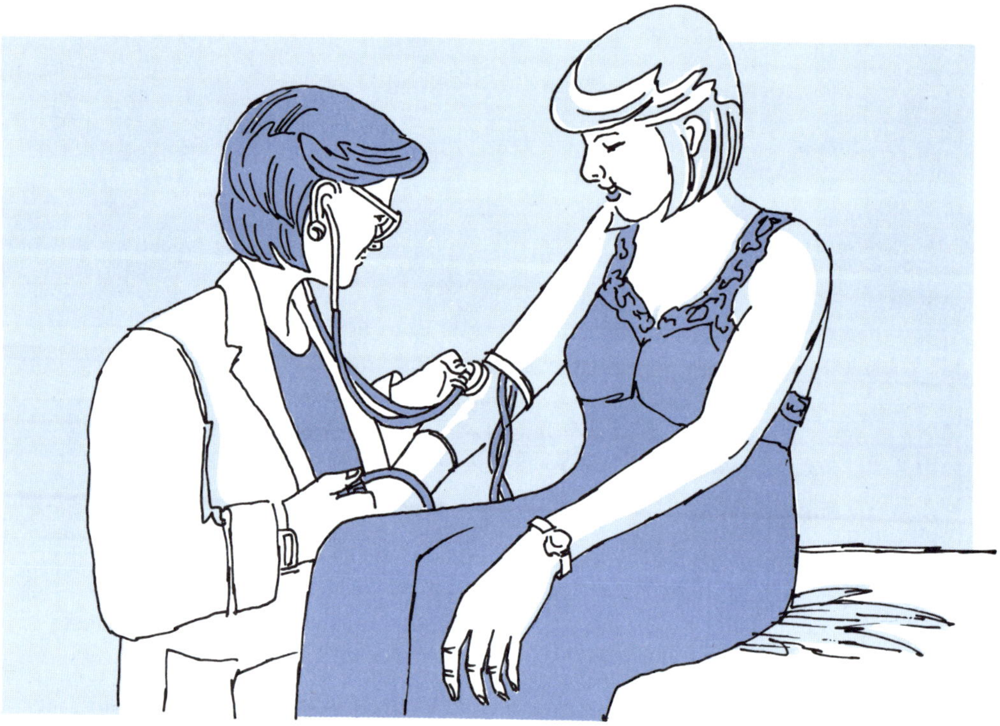

The menstrual cycle

When should your periods start?

There is tremendous, but normal, variation in when girls have their first period (known as menarche). The transformation from girl to woman involves a series of physical changes that occur over a number of years. The onset of periods actually occurs fairly late in that series of changes. As a rough guide, you can expect your periods to appear at least two years after your breasts have started to develop. Girls usually start to develop breasts some time between the ages of eight and thirteen years, with the majority showing some breast development by eleven years. It is quite usual to find that breasts develop unequally, one side being larger than the other. This may be embarrassing, but be reassured that the size will equalise in time. See tables on page 37 for more on development and maturity.

What will your periods be like?

It is equally normal for your periods to be irregular and light at the start, or quite heavy. Strenuous physical exercise and undernourishment can delay the onset of periods and can also cause menstrual irregularities. Many young girls also suffer from painful periods. We don't know why these differences occur between women, or how to influence them.

It is not so long ago that women in our society were protected and coddled while menstruating. Those days are now gone. Menstruation is a normal part of a woman's life, so continue with your activities as usual. Tampons have made activities, such as swimming and active sports, much easier to manage while menstruating.

What is 'normal'?

❑ ***Regularity*** Some perfectly healthy women menstruate as often as every three weeks and others only every few months. Both of these patterns and all those in between are perfectly normal. You should see your doctor if your menstrual cycle has changed for no apparent reason.

❑ ***How long and how heavy*** For some women, a period only lasts a couple of days, whereas others may experience a week of heavy bleeding. Various forms of contraception can affect your periods. The contraceptive pill is renowned for making your periods lighter and the intrauterine device for making periods heavier. Report any change in bleeding pattern to your doctor.

❑ ***Sex during menstruation*** There is no modern medical reason to prevent you having sex during your period. It's a matter of personal choice and comfort. You might like to discuss this with your partner.

❑ ***Painful periods*** There is medication to relieve severe pain during periods, such as the analgesics (pain relievers) paracetamol and aspirin, or antiprostaglandin drugs. Your doctor can also prescribe the contraceptive pill to decrease blood flow and unusual pain.

❑ ***Iron tablets*** It is certainly not necessary for all menstruating women to take iron tablets, though they are more prone to anaemic conditions than men. If your periods are continually heavy, anaemia can occur so you should discuss regular courses of iron tablets with your doctor.

❑ ***Colour of menstrual flow*** Sometimes menstrual blood can be bright red, at other times it is dark. Clots may also occur. All these variations are normal. The darker colour develops when the blood has spent longer in passing from the uterus to the outside.

❑ ***Tampons versus pads*** The main argument in favour of tampons is the greater convenience and comfort. However, there is a problem associated with their use – the condition known as toxic shock syndrome.

Unusual bleeding

Menopausal or post-menopausal women, whose period has been absent for six months, should see their doctor if they have any vaginal bleeding. Your doctor will want to exclude cancer as a possible cause.

What is toxic shock syndrome?

This is a rare but serious condition caused, it is believed, by toxic substances released by bacterial infection. The symptoms are varied and include high temperature, vomiting, diarrhoea, collapse and shock. Although it is associated with tampon usage, it can also occur after having a baby, or as a result of an infection under wounds. The person becomes very ill and requires emergency admission to hospital for intravenous antibiotics and fluids.

Reducing the risk of toxic shock

❑ Do not use tampons when you are unwell.

❑ Change your tampons frequently, every couple of hours, and preferably don't use them at night while you sleep.

❑ Change tampons each time you go to the toilet.

❑ Wash your hands well before and after changing the tampon.

❑ Remember to remove the tampon.

❑ Use tampons for convenience during sport and times of heavy flow, and pads at night.

❑ A new product, similar to a diaphragm, which holds a larger amount of menstrual blood, is also available.

A large number of girls and women would like to use tampons, but have difficulty inserting them. They are very uncomfortable if incorrectly inserted. Your doctor can help if this is a problem.

TAMPONS OR PADS

These days, many women prefer to use tampons for convenience sake. If you do choose tampons, be alert to the risk of toxic shock

Premenstrual tension (PMT)

Traditionally, premenstrual tension (PMT) refers to physical and psychological changes lasting a few days or a week before the onset of menstrual bleeding. By definition, the symptoms should cease with menstrual flow. Premenstrual tension does not affect all women. The number and variety of symptoms that are being attributed to premenstrual tension are considerable.

Physical symptoms can include breast discomfort, lower abdominal pain, a feeling of being bloated, changed bowel habits, weight gain and headache.

Psychological symptoms include anxiety, depression, irritability and inability to concentrate properly.

DO YOU HAVE PMT?

Do you have:

- ❑ Physical or psychological symptoms, such as those described on this page
- ❑ Do your symptoms appear about a week before your period and cease when it begins

What causes PMT?

At present, no-one really knows the cause of premenstrual tension but extensive research is being carried out. Hormonal changes and/or fluid retention seem to be the most commonly suggested culprits. Because we do not know the cause, treatments are directed to minimising the discomfort of the symptoms.

Some of these are:

- ❑ Diuretic medications to reduce fluid retention.
- ❑ Various vitamins. Traditionally, vitamin B1 has been used for breast symptoms, and vitamin B6 for depression and mood changes. These measures are not scientifically proven.
- ❑ Anti-prostaglandin medications as suggested by your doctor.
- ❑ Paying attention to your lifestyle, such as ensuring you are getting enough sleep, eating a balanced diet, and planning your schedule to avoid too much stress at your vulnerable times. Having some time to yourself is also helpful.

How do you know if it is stress or PMT?

Many women, suffering a variety of physical and psychological symptoms, have been confused about the cause of their problems. Very often they have not even been able to connect these various happenings. Sometimes, they are told by health professionals that they are simply suffering from stress. Keeping a calendar of your symptoms for two months before you attend your doctor can be helpful in sorting out the cause and identifying the problem as PMT.

A large number of women who accurately record their symptoms find that what they are calling premenstrual tension is in fact present all the time, but intensifies premenstrually. Many of them are women who spend their whole lives looking after others, spending little, if any, time satisfying their own needs. When these women make lifestyle changes, such as spending more time on themselves, exercising, relaxing and basically taking good quality time for themselves, their symptoms often decrease, or even disappear. Dietary changes, such as reducing salt, alcohol, cigarettes and caffeine use, may also help. However, this will not solve the problems of all premenstrual tension sufferers, and there will still be those who require medical supervision and treatment.

Dealing with stress

Identifying the problem as stress-related will not necessarily solve it. Many women may not feel in a position to make the necessary changes to reduce stress in their lives. Your doctor should be able to encourage you and suggest solutions. Some women receive the support they require from regular contact with a caring family doctor. Others require regular, more intensive psychiatric counselling. Your doctor will be able to refer you. There are courses available for self-assertion, and special support groups for women with similar problems. Learning to say 'no' to the demands of others may be a good way to begin dealing with the problem.

Menopause

Menopause refers to the time in a woman's life when her periods permanently cease.

This occurs as a result of age-related changes in the ovaries which now produce less oestrogen and progesterone. The age at which this may occur is variable. Some women reach menopause at the age of forty and others not until they are sixty. The average age is the late forties or early fifties. Your female relatives' experience of the menopause may give you an indication of what to expect. You certainly can't rely on this, but for many women it does hold true.

Surgical menopause occurs when both ovaries are removed before the normal change of life. Removal of only one ovary will not result in menopausal changes, because one healthy ovary is capable of producing sufficient hormones. The effects of surgical menopause are generally overcome by the prescription of replacement hormones in tablet form.

Climacteric or perimenopause refers to the time just before menopause – when symptoms or signs of approaching menopause may occur – and for at least twelve months after. Postmenopause is the term used to designate the time after the climacteric.

About a quarter of menopausal women will notice no symptoms at all, about half will notice some symptoms and another quarter will suffer quite severe problems

Symptoms of the menopause

The attention given to the menopause makes many women feel that they will all suffer problems, but this need not always be the case. In fact, you may experience a sense of wellbeing when no longer troubled by the fear of pregnancy.

As with all stages of life, there are certain age-related changes occurring at this time. Many women face the 'empty nest' syndrome when children leave home, and feel a sense of loss as a vacuum is left in their lives. They will need to find new interests to fill the void. There may also be an awareness of bodily ageing and a sense of loss that childbearing is no longer possible. It is not uncommon for a woman's parents and those of her husband to be entering an age of dependence, and often it is the woman who attends to their day-to-day care. Your own sense of mortality and grief at ageing becomes intensified. The problem is that many of these life crises become confused and are blamed on the physical changes of menopause.

Having said that, there are a number of physical changes that can occur. During menopause, about 25 per cent of women notice no changes, 50 per cent may notice some change and 25 per cent will experience very upsetting changes. You may experience none, some, or all of the following adverse symptoms.

❑ ***Hot flushes*** About 75 per cent of women may experience hot flushes around or after menopause. It is a feeling of warmth that occurs quickly over the body, most strongly on the face, neck and upper chest. Sweating occurs, and for some women it may be drenching, even awakening them at night. The exact cause is not known, but it is believed that the hormonal changes affect the blood vessels, making them open up temporarily on the skin surface.

❑ ***Pelvic changes*** The hormonal changes occurring in menopause cause the tissues lining the vagina and vulva to become thin. The pelvic muscles become more slack. These changes occur slowly over years and are sometimes accompanied by itchiness, discharge and urinary symptoms, due to similar changes in the urinary tract. This includes a sensation of burning on passing urine. Many women also notice that lubrication during sexual intercourse is decreased, so that sex becomes more uncomfortable.

❑ ***Breasts*** Breasts can become smaller.

❑ ***Bones*** Bones can become thinner (see the section on osteoporosis on page 43).

❑ ***Skin changes*** These may be blamed on hormonal changes, but don't forget that years of exposure to the elements and lack of skin care may also be taking their toll.

❏ ***Strokes and heart disease*** Before women enter the menopause they suffer these diseases less than men do. Once a woman passes the age of menopause the occurrence of these diseases is similar to that in men.

❏ ***Behavioural changes*** Some women may develop nervous changes such as depression, anxiety and irritability. One theory is that these women may become more vulnerable to other stresses, due to hormonal changes. 'Menopausal madness' is now regarded as a myth but, unfortunately, many women have been told by their mothers or grandmothers that insanity is connected with the menopause. This myth is definitely untrue, but continues to haunt some women who are too scared or embarrassed to consult their doctor.

CONTRACEPTION AFTER MENOPAUSE

❏ Do not rely on decreasing fertility to prevent pregnancy as you approach menopause

❏ If you are younger than fifty years when your menopause occurs, you should use contraceptive measures for two years after your last period

❏ If you are over fifty years at menopause, you should use additional contraception for one year

Treatment of the menopause

Oestrogen is the mainstay of treatment for the menopausal symptoms. It cannot be taken by some women who have a history of deep venous thrombosis, liver or gall bladder disease, or a past history of certain cancers. The presence of other factors such as increased blood pressure, high blood fats and diabetes also needs to be carefully considered before hormones are prescribed.

❏ ***Hot flushes*** Oestrogen is taken in tablet form for approximately three weeks every month. In addition, a second hormone called progesterone is added to protect the womb from changes that could lead to cancer.
For women who choose not to or who cannot take oestrogen, a doctor might prescribe a small dose of clonidine.

❏ ***Pelvic changes*** Your doctor may prescribe oestrogen tablets to take orally or an oestrogen-containing cream to be applied directly to the vaginal area.

❏ ***Mood changes*** Oestrogen may or may not actually affect mood. Some studies suggest that it does, particularly in women who have other symptoms of hormonal deficiency, such as hot flushes. Whether it is the removal of the distressing physical symptoms that makes you feel better, or whether there is an actual effect on mood by the hormone itself, is not really known.

❏ ***Skin*** There is no evidence that oestrogen will make you more youthful.

❏ ***Bones*** Oestrogen is being actively promoted as a method for preventing the bone loss of osteoporosis. (See the section on osteoporosis on page 43.)

CHANGES DURING MENOPAUSE

Psychosocial Changes	Physical Changes
'Empty nest' syndrome	Hot flushes
Awareness of bodily ageing	Breasts can become smaller
Care and responsibility of parents	Pelvic changes – itchiness, discharge, urinary symptoms
Mood changes	Bones become thinner
Behavioural changes due to depression, anxiety and irritability	Skin changes

Osteoporosis

In osteoporosis the bone becomes thinner, but still keeps the normal mineral content. Osteoporotic bone is weaker and breaks more easily than normal bone. You may not know you have osteoporosis until a bone breaks. About a quarter of menopausal women will develop osteoporosis.

WHO IS AT RISK?

Women at greater risk are those who:

- are lighter
- exercise less
- have a family history of osteoporosis
- smoke
- go through the menopause early
- have had period of amenorrhoea (no periods)
- drink a lot of alcohol
- are on steroids
- drink more than five cups of coffee per day

Why does it happen? The fall in hormone levels in postmenopausal women seems to be linked to a thinning of bones. Men have a much more gradual age-related thinning of bones. Some doctors believe fervently in the need for most women to take hormone therapy plus increased calcium around the time of the menopause. They argue that osteoporosis is the direct result of the lack of hormone. Other doctors are concerned about as yet unknown side effects of this treatment. Every woman in this age group should discuss the pros and cons of therapy before embarking on treatment. The role played by diet is also under scrutiny. A lot of protein or salt and not enough calcium in the diet can lower calcium levels, contributing to the condition.

Detecting osteoporosis

It is only when the bones are down to about 50 per cent of their original density that osteoporosis can be detected on X-ray. A fracture is usually the first sign. Another sign that osteoporosis is developing is loss of height – elderly folk do, in fact, shrink with age, producing the humped back known as 'dowager's hump'. The bones most likely to be affected are in the back. They often collapse without pain, and this may only be detected on X-ray. A collapsed vertebra can also be extremely painful. Other bones that commonly break are the wrist, the pelvis and the hip.

There are tests being developed to try and identify the women most likely to develop the disease. If this can be done, those who would most benefit from hormonal treatment can be given it before any fractures occur. A machine to measure bone density has recently been developed. It is designed to predict those most likely to develop osteoporosis, as well as monitoring treatment. Unfortunately it is not generally available at the moment.

Prevention

Adequate calcium should be included in the diet from an early age.
Foods that contain large amounts of calcium include dairy products, some fish (particularly tinned ones, complete with bone), chick peas, soya beans, tofu, miso, seaweed, almonds, brazil nuts, hazelnuts and blackstrap molasses. Certain green vegetables such as parsley, chives and broccoli have a reasonable amount of calcium as do sesame and sunflower seeds.

Decreasing alcohol, cigarette and caffeine intake can also help reduce your chances of developing the condition. If you also require a low cholesterol diet you might need to be cautious with dairy products and obtain most of your calcium requirement from the other sources.

The prevention of osteoporosis is yet another reason to exercise. Weight-bearing exercise is more effective in building up and maintaining bone mass in osteoporotic bone than non-weight-bearing exercise.

SUGGESTED DAILY CALCIUM INTAKE

Infants	360 mg
Children	800 mg
Girls	1100-1700 mg
Adults	
men:	800 mg
women:	800-1000 mg
women at menopause:	1500 mg

OSTEOPOROSIS TREATMENT

Hormone replacement therapy is the main treatment available at present. This involves taking oestrogen (and progesterone as well if the womb is still present) together with calcium to decrease further bone loss. Other hormones known as anabolic agents can be prescribed for women who can't take oestrogen. Current research in this area may well offer new solutions

TYPICAL HORMONE SCHEDULE

A typical HRT schedule
- oestrogen days 1 to 24 of each calendar month
- progesterone days 12 to 24 of each calendar month
- nil days 24 to end of the month

Hormonal replacement therapy (HRT)

Two different types of hormone are generally given in hormone replacement therapy (HRT). The first is oestrogen, which used to be given alone until it was recognised that its use was associated with a higher incidence of cancer of the womb. There is some argument as to whether it should be given alone to women who have had hysterectomies. Women who still have a womb are given oestrogen and, for seven to ten days, a second hormone called progesterone to protect the womb from cancer.

There is no one correct way of giving hormones. Many women are confused about their hormone schedule. Basically, oestrogen should be given cyclically, with about one week's break every month or three weeks. Progesterone should be added to the oestrogen for at least the last twelve or so days each cycle.

In the case of a woman who has had a hysterectomy, oestogen generally would be given every day. Progesterone may or may not be added.

HORMONE SCHEDULE

Days of the month
1 2 4 6 8 10 12 14 16 18 20 22 24 26 28 30

Oestrogen Nil

Progesterone Nil

Hormonal replacement therapy (HRT) and periods

Some women will have withdrawal bleeding during that part of the cycle in which they are taking no hormones. Many of these women find this bleeding stops after being on HRT for about a year.

Administering oestrogen Currently, oestrogen is taken by mouth, intravaginal cream or pessary. There is research into new ways of taking hormones, either by implanting the hormone under the skin or by the use of a skin patch which releases the hormone through the skin. At present some heart medications are given by skin patch. These developments may mean that women who could not previously take hormones will be able to do so.

When to see your doctor

If you want to try HRT, see your doctor a few years before the menopause is likely to occur. If you are on HRT it is absolutely imperative that you consult your doctor if you notice any new bleeding.

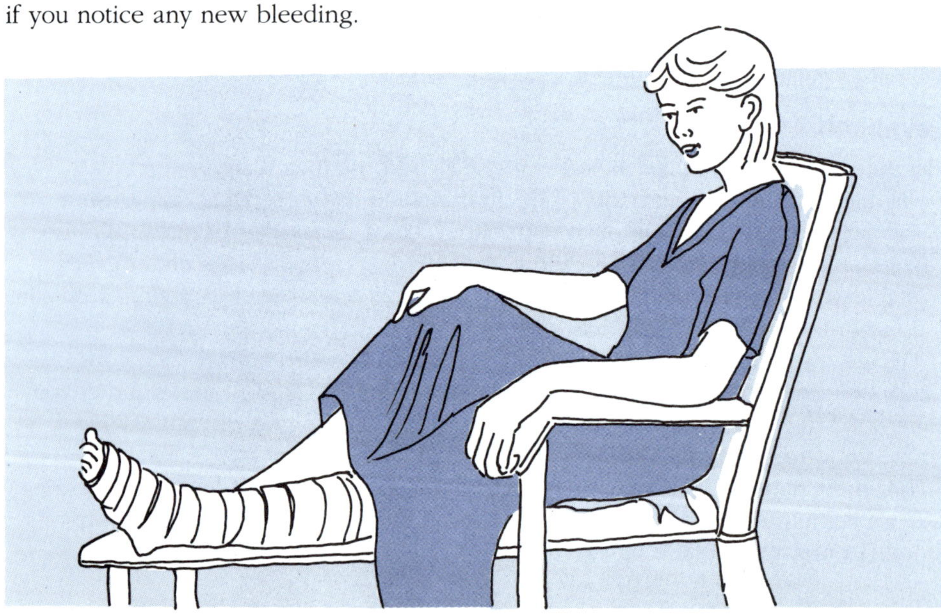

Incontinence

About six per cent of people probably suffer from incontinence, but only about one-third of them will have told their doctors. Unfortunately, incontinence is one of those subjects which the embarrassed sufferers are reluctant to talk about. Women are seven or eight times more likely to suffer incontinence than men. As many as a third of adult women can expect to experience this unpleasant problem at some time.

There are five main types of incontinence

❑ ***Stress incontinence*** where coughing, sneezing, exercising, straining or lifting causes urine to escape. This can be embarrassing and inhibit lifestyle, even though only small amounts of urine are lost.

❑ ***Dribble incontinence*** where leakage of urine occurs without obvious provocation.

❑ ***Overflow incontinence*** where the bladder fails to empty completely, resulting in chronic distension.

❑ ***Urge incontinence*** where overactive bladder contractions cause urine to leak before you can reach a toilet.

❑ ***Flooding incontinence*** where the overactive bladder contractions cause the whole contents of the bladder to be lost.

What can you do about stress incontinence?

Learning and practising pelvic muscle strengthening exercises can go a long way to prevent stress incontinence and can even rectify minor abnormality. For too many years we have ignored these important exercises. Instead of waiting until after childbearing, when symptoms become obvious, young girls should practise pelvic floor exercises as part of a regular fitness routine.

If you suffer from incontinence that your doctor believes requires further treatment, there are treatments and surgical procedures available. There have been many developments enabling more accurate diagnosis and treatment of this often hidden problem.

If you do suffer from incontinence do not hesitate to discuss the problem with your doctor. There are solutions available

Pelvic floor exercises Firstly, draw in your muscles as if you were going to stop yourself urinating. Check that you are using the correct muscles by actually stopping your flow of urine. Do this check only once on a couple of occasions; don't make a habit of it.

Secondly, practise tightening the muscles around the vaginal opening. You can check whether you've done this correctly by placing one or two clean fingers in the opening. If you are doing this exercise correctly, you will feel the squeeze on your fingers each time you tighten the muscles.

Thirdly, tighten the muscles around the anus, as if you were trying to stop yourself from passing wind. Hold this position for four or five seconds then release. Finally, combine all these exercises in one. Tighten all the muscles we have discussed and hold for a few seconds, relax for twenty seconds and then repeat.

Your doctor should be able to provide you with a more detailed explanation if you need one. Alternatively, consult a specially trained physiotherapist who teaches pelvic floor exercises.

How often should you do the exercises? Aim to do each of these exercises a couple of times a day, building them naturally into your day. A good way to remember them is to link them up with other activities, perhaps do one when you are stopped at a red light or as you clean your teeth.

Healthy pelvic tone helps in childbirth and improves sex life. Belly dancing incorporates pelvic toning in its technique, and could be a fun way to learn and practise this form of muscle exercise!

Hysterectomy

Hysterectomy is the most commonly performed major operation. It refers to the operation in which the womb is removed, because of physical disease, such as fibroids, endometriosis, pelvic infection, cancer, severe menorrhagia and, more rarely, after damage resulting from childbirth.

❑ ***Fibroids*** Up to one-third of women will have fibroids. These are just lumps of normal tissue in the wall of the uterus. Often they require no treatment, but if fibroids are causing symptoms, or growing rapidly, it is usual to remove them.

❑ ***Endometriosis*** This is a disease in which the tissue which normally lines the womb grows in other parts of the body, for example on the wall of the womb, tubes, ovaries. Many women live their lives totally unaware they have the condition. Others suffer extreme pain and even infertility. The disease sometimes disappears spontaneously but troublesome endometriosis can be treated with hormones, a drug called Danazol or surgery. Surgery can be conservative, to preserve fertility, or radical, involving hysterectomy.

❑ ***Pelvic infection*** Pelvic infection is common, but hysterectomy as a means of treating the infection is not. It is only in extremely severe, recurrent infections, where other methods have failed, that surgery is an option.

❑ ***Cancer*** About 3 per cent of women may develop a cancer of the uterus, tubes or ovaries. Surgical removal of the cancerous organs is then necessary. Which organs are removed will depend on the site and extent of the cancer.

❑ ***Accidental perforation*** Often the body will repair a small hole in the womb, caused during an operation or childbirth. Rarely, a hysterectomy may be needed.

❑ ***Prolapse*** The surgeon sometimes advises a hysterectomy be performed as part of a prolapse repair to improve the outcome of the surgery.

❑ ***Menorrhagia*** This condition of heavy, painful periods, causes a number of women to finally choose hysterectomy.

In some societies, preventive hysterectomy is undertaken to avoid any problems such as cancer, menstrual problems, or the need for contraception. The possible complications of surgery, time, cost and pain need to be balanced against this. Many women would find preventive hysterectomy repugnant, in principle.

Every woman should discuss the pros and cons of elective hysterectomy with her doctor, before embarking on surgery

Types of hysterectomy

There are a few different types of operation performed.

❑ ***Total hysterectomy*** The most common form of the operation, involving the removal of the whole womb.

❑ ***Subtotal hysterectomy*** Involves removal of the womb but not the cervix.

❑ ***Salpingo-oophorectomy*** This is the name given to the operation if the tubes and ovaries are also removed.

❑ ***Wertheim's extended hysterectomy*** Where not only the uterus, but also part of the vagina and other pelvic tissues are removed. This operation is required for some forms of cancer.

It is possible to perform a hysterectomy through the vagina or the abdomen. The latter is the more usual, and it is best to be guided by your surgeon.

Before undergoing an elective hysterectomy, make sure you understand what is involved. As with any operation, you have every right to make sure you have confidence in your surgeon before you decide to undergo an operation. Your family doctor should be your ally in this. If you are not satisfied with the options or explanations you have been given, discuss this with your family doctor. You can be referred to a second specialist should you want another opinion. This applies particularly if you are undergoing a nonessential or elective hysterectomy, rather than an essential one for cancer. If you are confused by different opinions, return to discuss them with your family doctor to help you make up your mind.

Coping with hysterectomy

As with any operation, the potential for complications is always there. Damage to the uterus, bladder, ureter and rectum have occurred in the past. Bleeding, infection and clots can also occur. Pneumonia and vaginal discharges can develop. Death is uncommon, occurring in one in every one thousand to three thousand operations. The elderly, and those who have medical conditions such as high blood pressure, cancer and obesity are more likely to be at risk.

Hysterectomy is a stressful operation. It is best to enter the operation well prepared. Many women are understandably concerned about the effect hysterectomy may have on their sex lives and appearance. There are many myths around causing women to believe that they will become less attractive and age more rapidly after hysterectomy. This is not the case. Just over half of a group of women surveyed in Sydney (Australia) reported improved sexual relationships after the operation. Not unexpectedly, couples with other psychological or relationship problems are more likely to experience problems after hysterectomy. Be reassured that there is no reason for you to age early or for your skin to wrinkle and become dry suddenly just because you've had a hysterectomy. For many women, a hysterectomy that removes years of painful symptoms can give a positive feeling of wellbeing.

If you need help in the postoperative period, your doctor or local community health centre may be able to advise you if a self-help group exists locally.

Most women are fearful of the prospect of hysterectomy. However, the cessation of unpleasant or painful symptoms and the freedom from the fear of unwanted pregnancy, can in fact lead to a very positive result

Other problems

Prolapse

It is common for women as they age, particularly if they have borne children, to suffer a certain degree of prolapse, when the uterus falls a little in relation to the surrounding tissue. In addition, the walls of the rectum (behind the vagina) may weaken to form a rectocele, or the wall of the urethra or bladder in front of the vagina may weaken, ballooning into the vagina to form a cysto-urethrocele. If the uterus falls sufficiently, you may feel an unpleasant dragging sensation. Bladder or bowel symptoms, including incontinence, may develop if the walls of the urinary system or rectal system weaken (see section on Incontinence on page 45).

Vaginismus

This is a condition in which the muscles surrounding the vagina go into spasm, making sexual intercourse difficult or impossible. See your doctor if this should occur. Sometimes inflammation or some other physical condition can be responsible. Often underlying problems or emotional reasons underlie the condition, such as previous sexual violence, fear of pregnancy and so on. If this is the case, sexual counselling is available. Each situation needs to be assessed individually. A carefully supervised program of gradual stimulation and the insertion of vaginal dilators of increasing size, or an increasing number of fingers, can often cure the condition.

Retroverted uterus

The uterus can lie in a number of different positions. If it is rotated forwards it is described as anteversion and if it is rotated backwards it is a retroversion. In some cases, it can move from one position to another. Retroversion is much like being left-handed rather than right-handed! The main myth associated with retroversion is that it is associated with infertility. Don't believe it – generally you are just as likely to become pregnant whichever way your uterus lies.

Cervical cancer

Cervical cancer is one of the killers of women in developed countries. Tragically, it is avoidable. Early detection and treatment of cervical cancer by regular cervical/PAP smear tests are essential. For this test, your doctor will remove a few cells from the cervix for microscopic examination. Many of the deaths from cervical cancer occur in women who have never attended for a cervical/PAP smear test, because of ignorance and lack of information.

The cervical/PAP smear test

Before invasive cancer, with its attendant death rate, occurs there is a series of changes that can be picked up. If these changes are adequately treated there is no risk of developing invasive cancer. These changes cause no symptoms. Regular cervical/PAP smear tests will identify these changes. After treatment, you must continue to have regular smear tests as the condition may recur.

How often should you have a smear test? Most authorities recommend a smear test every year and all experts agree that one should be taken at least every three years providing you have had a few clear ones and no new risk factors. Remembering something each year is easier, because you can link it to some other event, for example, Christmas, the start of winter, your birthday or an anniversary.

Who should have a cervical/PAP smear test? All women who have been, or are, sexually active should have regular smear tests. You should have a smear test within twelve months of beginning a sexual relationship. Women over sixty-five years do not need to be tested if they have had at least two recent smear tests and no abnormal smear tests in the preceding ten years.

Smear tests and hysterectomy It used to be thought that a cervical/PAP smear test was not necessary after a hysterectomy, because you are most unlikely to still have a cervix. These days a smear test is taken from the vaginal vault (a vaginal vault smear test). It is not as necessary to have this type of smear test as often – every five years is considered adequate. However, a pelvic examination to exclude any masses or palpable cancer should still be done every year. If you have had a subtotal hysterectomy and still have a cervix you should continue to have smear tests every twelve to eighteen months.

What causes cervical cancer?

It is not known exactly what causes cervical cancer. However, it is known that certain behaviour or conditions are more likely to result in the development of this disease. Firstly, it appears that the disease only occurs in women who have had sexual intercourse. This observation has led to the theory that the male may be transmitting some factor in the sperm or a virus or some other chemical associated with his lifestyle. It has also been noted that women who have sex earlier and with more partners are more likely to develop the disease. Research is also looking at her male partner's sexual behaviour as a factor in a woman developing cervical cancer.

Other factors associated with the disease include smoking and possibly the Pill. Smoking may affect the development of cancer of the cervix, because its by-products concentrate in the cervical cells. The possible association with the Pill means that women on the Pill should make doubly sure that they have regular smear tests.

Another factor that has been associated with the development of cervical cancer is the presence of the 'wart' virus, which has been found in large numbers of cervical precancers. It is not proved whether the presence of the warts is the cause of the abnormal cells, or whether the abnormal cells are a more comfortable environment for the wart virus. However, the warts are contagious, and if present should be treated. The wart virus can be present and passed on to others without causing any visible lesions. Although a sexually transmitted method is our current understanding of the relationship between the wart virus and cervical cancer, not all cases can be explained in this way.

AVOIDING CERVICAL CANCER

- Have regular cervical/PAP smear tests and remember to check up on the results
- Stop smoking
- Use condoms if you have any casual sexual encounters or new sexual partners
- Avoid sex, or use condoms, with known or suspected genital wart sufferers. Condoms and diaphragms will reduce sperm contact, which seems to be crucial in developing the disease

Medical procedures

If your smear test shows precancerous changes, you will be sent for a colposcopy examination. The colposcope is a special type of magnifying instrument which provides the doctor with a good view of changes in your cervix. A biopsy can also be done if needed.

If your doctor decides further treatment is necessary, the cells will need to be removed. One of the latest methods for doing this is by laser beam under either a local or a general anaesthetic. Other methods used include electrocoagulation diathermy in which the cells are burned off with an electric current or a cone biopsy in which a triangular segment of the abnormal and surrounding cells is removed.

The cure rate of these procedures is excellent. The abnormality may recur in about two per cent of cases – so follow-up is essential. A postoperative check is usually done three to four weeks after the procedure and then regular cervical/PAP smear tests and colposcopy. In order to decrease the death rate associated with this preventable disease, it is absolutely essential that all women aged less than sixty-five years who are or have been sexually active attend their doctor regularly for a cervical/PAP smear test.

Breast cancer

One in sixteen women will develop breast cancer and one in twenty-four will die from the disease. The risk increases where there is a close family history of breast cancer. Early detection of breast cancer is crucial to effective treatment and the long-term survival of the patient. More than ninety per cent of patients whose breast cancer is detected early, survive the first five years after treatment. This is the generally accepted point at which doctors will speak in terms of cure. Early detection ensures that the disease is arrested while it is still localised within the breast and, hopefully, within a small area of the breast.

Detecting breast cancer

The best insurance against the most serious effects of breast cancer is regular self-examination. Unfortunately, only a small percentage of women regularly examine their own breasts. Ideally, you should examine each breast carefully once a month, about a week after your period. This will ensure that you are not confused by hormonal changes which occur in the breasts during the menstrual cycle. It is very important that you become familiar with the normal contours of your breast. In this way you will notice any change when it occurs. Your doctor will show you the best technique for breast self-examination.

Another method of detecting tumours in the breast is by mammography. This is a form of X-ray which identifies changes. This procedure, which is quite costly, may in future be available to all women as a screening procedure.

Treating breast cancer

There are a number of surgical procedures available to treat breast cancer. Which one is chosen depends on the extent of the cancer as well as your general health.

- A partial mastectomy in which breast tissue and glands from the armpit are removed.
- A simple mastectomy in which only the breast tissue is removed.
- A radical mastectomy where not only breast tissue and glands are removed, but chest muscle as well. This operation is now quite rare.
- A lumpectomy where only the actual lump and some surrounding tissue are removed.

Surgical procedures are often combined with other forms of treatment such as chemotherapy and deep X-ray. In addition, your doctor may advise treatment by a physiotherapist. Your doctor and surgeon will choose the most appropriate treatment for you. Remember, you are always entitled to a second opinion.

Men's health issues are often forgotten. By covering the more intimate areas of medical problems, it is hoped that men will realise that they too can discuss problems or queries with their doctor.

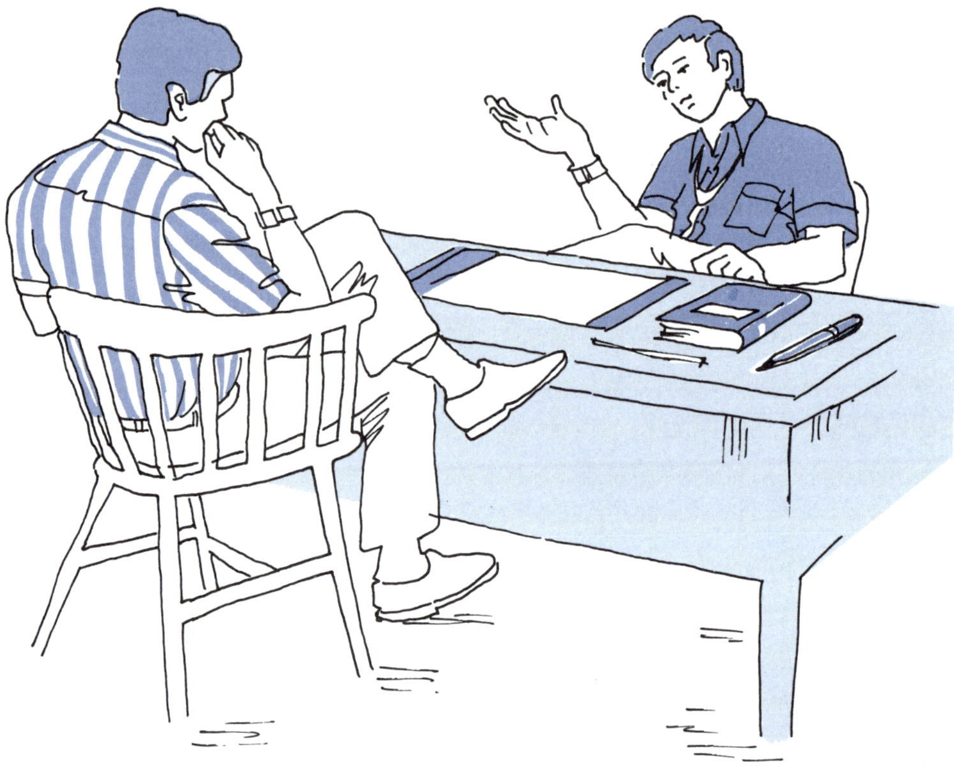

Diseases of the prostate

The prostate gland is a small gland which lies beneath the bladder in men. Its function is to produce part of the seminal fluid.

All men over the age of fifty years should have their prostate gland checked by their family doctor. This test involves an assessment of the size and consistency of the prostate, by a doctor performing a manual examination through the rectum.

- ***Prostatitis*** This is often caused by a bacterial infection, involving an underlying urinary or sexually transmitted infection, causing the prostate gland to become inflamed. Symptoms that indicate the possible presence of an infection include painful and frequent urination, an unpleasant odour, urine that shows the presence of blood, fever and back pain. Treatment includes administration of antibiotics and adequate intake of fluids, as well as attention to any underlying abnormality.
- ***Enlarged prostate*** As men age, the prostate gland may become enlarged. Symptoms of enlargement may be experienced as the gland presses on the bladder and urethra. A man with an enlarged prostate may notice that he needs to go to the toilet more frequently at night, that the urine stream may be slow to start, and dribbling may occur. Sometimes he may feel that his bladder is not quite empty when he has finished his urination. In addition, erections of the penis may be painful.

Although the doctor is mindful of the occurrence of prostate cancer when faced with any of the above symptoms, in most cases the enlargement of the prostate is not due to cancer.

❑ ***Prostate cancer*** The cause of prostate cancer is not known although it is one of the more common cancers affecting men. The occurrence of this type of cancer is gradually increasing. The older a man is the more likely he is to develop the condition. This form of cancer is not often seen in men younger than fifty, but it occasionally does occur in this age group. Early diagnosis and treatment are vital.

Treatment Treatment of prostate cancer involves surgery. Depending on the stage the cancer has reached, the testes may also need to be removed. If this does prove to be necessary, replacement hormones may be prescribed.

Benign enlargement of the prostate that causes symptoms severe enough to warrant treatment, involves an operation in which the prostate is removed. The removal takes place through the urethra. There is a new medication available to help decrease symptoms for a few weeks while awaiting surgery.

PROSTATE PROBLEMS	
You may have an infection in the prostate gland	**You may have an enlarged prostate gland**
if your urine ❑ is painful and frequent ❑ has an unpleasant odour ❑ is dark reddish-brown (presence of blood)	if your urine ❑ is slow to start ❑ is dribbling
and you experience ❑ fever ❑ backache	and you experience ❑ feeling of fullness of bladder after urination ❑ painful erections of the penis ❑ constant need to go to toilet
Treatment commonly involves ❑ antibiotics ❑ greater intake of fluids ❑ attention to any underlying abnormality	Treatment commonly involves ❑ may involve operation to remove prostate ❑ medication for a few weeks while awaiting surgery

Diseases of the testes

A normal male has two testes. Each one is located in a scrotal sac. From puberty onwards the testes produce sperm cells and male sex hormones. For further information see the table on genital maturity in the Children's section on page 37.

❑ ***Orchitis*** This term refers to inflammation of the testis, caused by a bacteria or a virus, for example in mumps. Mumps orchitis can result in infertility. In this case the infection cannot be treated with antibiotics as they have no effect on viral infection.

Sexually transmitted diseases may also cause orchitis.

❑ ***Torsion of the testis*** This is a painful condition where a testis has become twisted. Shock can develop and an emergency operation is needed to disentangle the torsion ensuring, at the same time, that the blood supply to the testis is not cut off.

❑ ***Undescended testis*** The testis travels from the abdomen to the scrotum during the inter-utero development of the male foetus. At birth, it is common for one or both testes to have not fully completed their descent into the scrotal cavity. Sometimes the descent will be completed in early babyhood. If not, treatment may be needed. Treatment with hormones or surgery can be used to bring the testis down. If the testes are allowed to remain in the abdomen, infertility will result.

SEXUAL PROBLEMS

Achieving a satisfying sexual relationship is a great concern to many people, often expressed in anxiety about performance. This anxiety is frequently the greatest sexual problem.

Because sexual functioning has so many complex emotional and social implications, it has become fraught with misconceptions, confusion and unhappiness. Our society regards itself as having a 'liberated' attitude to sex, yet myths still abound.

It would be impossible to list all the anxieties associated with sexuality. The human mind is most inventive when it comes to creating problems and anxieties! The most common worry is probably 'am I normal?'. Remember, there is a tremendous variation in what is 'normal' sexual behaviour – just about everything that you and your partner are comfortable with is perfectly all right.

Many people worry that they have a problem in sexual appetite or performance, because they have 'read something somewhere'. Often all that is needed is reassurance or some basic information. Your doctor can also identify anything that needs more specific counselling.

How often is it normal to have sex?

There is no defined 'norm' in sexual frequency. Some couples may have sexual intercourse every day, other couples once a month. The most important thing is that both partners in the relationship are happy with the arrangement.

What is satisfactory sex?

This question usually involves anxiety about orgasm. So much has been written about mutual orgasm that many people consider this the hallmark of so-called 'satisfactory sex'. This is not the case. Some people can experience a satisfying sexual relationship without orgasm. The real measure of a satisfactory sexual relationship between two people is whether both are satisfied. There is no need to compare or measure performance with the experience of others.

Is masturbation normal?

Masturbation is a healthy, normal sexual outlet. Even small children can derive pleasure and security from touching themselves. It is appropriate to accept masturbation as normal and to teach children that although it is acceptable, it is private, and should not be practised in front of others.

When are you too old for sex?

While procreation is no longer possible, there is no cut-off point at which age sex should cease. Many elderly couples continue to enjoy a sexual relationship. There can be a number of advantages associated with advancing age and sex. The fear of an unwanted pregnancy has gone as has the pressure to perform – a common worry of the younger man. Privacy and time are more easily available than during a younger, more active stage of life.

With advancing age, sexual arousal can take longer, and after the hormonal changes of menopause, some women find sex painful. This may be caused by the thinner, more fragile lining of the vagina.

Treatment with hormones, either in the form of a local cream or by mouth, can help. Continued sexual activity is also believed to be beneficial in the prevention of the condition.

Who can help you?

For many people with a sexual problem, their first call will be to their general practitioner or family planning centre. Ask for referral to a trained sex therapist if that is what you prefer. Remember, there is always help available.

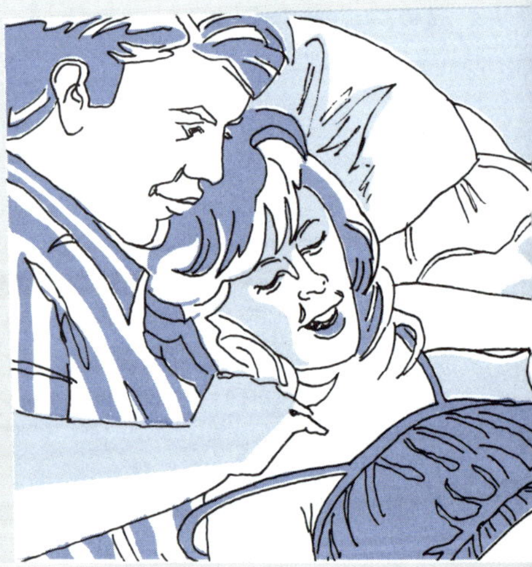

Male sexual problems

Many men just need reassurance that techniques are available which may help their problem.

Responding to sexual counselling often requires learning new techniques. However, like learning to ride a bicycle, these new techniques require perseverance and practice in order to achieve success. 'Instant' solutions to this problem are rare – effort is often required.

Sexual problems in relationships often involve problems in both the sexual and the emotional area. Some emotional problems will appear to be sexual problems and vice versa. In many cases the two have become pretty mixed up together by the time a man, woman or couple asks for help.

Premature ejaculation

This problem may be present from the earliest sexual experiences or it may develop later in life, following a period of good ejaculatory control. In the first instance, the man has failed to learn how to control his ejaculation. Anxiety, lack of knowledge and inexperience all contribute to the problem. You can learn and practise specific exercises to control ejaculation, either alone or with a sexual partner. Your doctor can advise you or refer you to a specialist/ therapist for help if necessary.

In the second case, normal ejaculatory functioning ceases. It is important that your doctor eliminates any physical factors that could be responsible for the change in ejaculation.

Ask your doctor for advice.

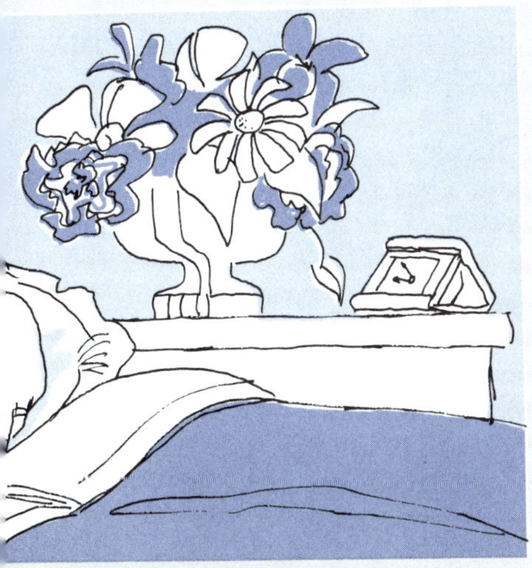

Impotence

Impotence refers to a man's inability to achieve and maintain an erection in order to have sexual intercourse. There are many causes for this condition. These can be divided into psychological and physical causes and often both areas contribute to the problem. Certain prescribed medications can also contribute to a man's impotence.

Treatment Experience in dealing with these problems is needed to elicit the underlying reasons for their occurrence. See your doctor and discuss the problem without embarrassment. Your doctor may refer you to someone especially skilled in this area for further advice and counselling.

There are also physical treatments available for problems diagnosed as physical ones. These include the self-injection of drugs to increase blood flow, special vacuum pumps to raise an erection, surgery in some cases and an inflatable prosthesis. The use of these measures is very specific and must be appropriately prescribed by a specialist practitioner. General counselling will help to overcome anxiety. Specific counselling from a sex therapist can be directed towards learning techniques for increasing sexual responsiveness.

Achieving a satisfactory sexual relationship

It is commonly believed that a man should know how to satisfy a woman. This kind of myth puts incredible pressure on men. It is quite untrue. Neither partner can be assured that they will automatically know what turns their partner on. Each of us is unique. Some like to be stimulated in one way, others in another way. Sexual interaction is like communication. Both verbal and nonverbal communication can assist you in identifying ways of increasing sexual pleasure for yourself and your partner. You don't have a special sense to tell you how to satisfy your partner – ask !

Penis size The ability to have a satisfying sexual relationship is not usually dependent on the size of your penis.

Many men and boys are concerned about the size of their penis. There is a normal variation in the size of the flaccid penis, but the size of the erect penis is not as variable. Putting aside such anxieties is a positive step towards achieving a happy relationship.

Having a baby is an important milestone in your life. In one step, you and your partner move from being a couple to being a family, with all its attendant problems and pleasures. Paying attention to good health practices will help to ensure a healthy pregnancy and a good start for your baby.

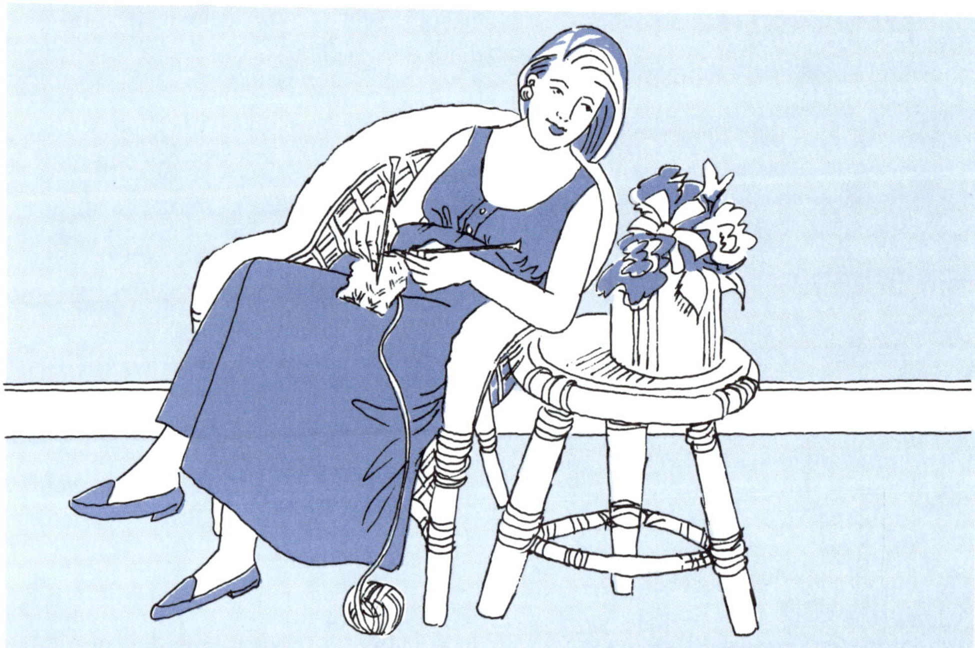

Pregnancy

Ideally, preparing for pregnancy should start before conception. Women are increasingly aware of this and are seeking pre-pregnancy advice. One way in which you can prepare for pregnancy is in paying attention to lifestyle factors which can affect your own health or your baby's. These factors include diet, exercise and avoiding all drugs including alcohol and nicotine. One important test your doctor can perform for you before you become pregnant, is to find out if you are immune to German measles (rubella). It is wise to be sure you are immune before you become pregnant. This certainly diminishes the anxiety you will feel should you inadvertently come into contact with German measles while pregnant. If your blood test shows that you are not immune to German measles, you can be immunised and retested three months later. It is important that you do not become pregnant for three months after the injection. Hopefully, we will see a drop in the rate of occurrence of German measles with the new vaccination policies in force. When you begin pregnancy fit, relaxed and healthy, it is a bonus for your baby.

Antenatal care

It is only since early this century that so much attention has been focused on the pregnant woman and, even more recently, on her partner. The aim of antenatal care is to make sure that a healthy mother has a healthy baby. As soon as you suspect you are pregnant, visit your doctor, confirm the pregnancy and make arrangements for your antenatal care.

What will your doctor need to know? Your doctor needs to know your medical history and present level of health. Throughout your pregnancy, your weight is monitored to check how much you gain over what period of time. Your doctor will also check your blood pressure and your urine. You will be observed to see if you are retaining fluids. At various stages in the pregnancy, blood tests are done to detect any pregnancy-related illness.

Special tests

- ***Ultrasound*** Ultrasound provides an image of the baby in the uterus. It does not use X-rays, but high frequency sound waves. The technique is most commonly used to monitor the size of the baby. It can also tell you if you are carrying more than one baby and if the placenta is in the right position.
- ***Chorionic villus biopsy*** This is a relatively new test, performed as early as eight to ten weeks into the pregnancy, to detect Down's syndrome or other chromosomal abnormalities. There is a certain risk of miscarriage with this procedure, but as our skill develops, the rate is decreasing. The advantage is that a result is available earlier than with the more traditional method of amniocentesis.
- ***Amniocentesis*** Around the sixteenth week of pregnancy, a sample of amniotic fluid is collected for testing. This test also detects Down's syndrome and other chromosomal abnormalities. It can also tell you the sex of the baby – if you want to know. It takes a few weeks to get the results, and is not without risk.

These two tests – chorionic villus biopsy and amniocentesis – are usually reserved for women over the age of thirty-five years or women already identified as having a high risk of producing an abnormal baby.

Looking after yourself

- ***Smoking*** As a parent, you are well advised to be a nonsmoker. Smokers are more likely to have smaller babies, miscarry, produce a stillborn infant and have complicated births. Children living in a smoking environment are less healthy and develop more respiratory infections.
- ***Alcohol*** This is another drug best avoided during pregnancy. Fortunately, a number of women find that they no longer enjoy alcohol when pregnant. Babies born to heavy drinkers can suffer from a syndrome called fetal alcohol syndrome (FAS), which is associated with a number of abnormalities. No one can be sure if there is a safe level of alcohol intake for the unborn child. Total abstinence is wise.
- ***Medication*** Before taking any medication, talk to your doctor. Many drugs are not safe during pregnancy. If you are on permanent medication, discuss this with your doctor when planning your pregnancy. It is often essential that medicines taken for chronic diseases are continued during pregnancy.

Don't assume that any doctor you see knows that you are pregnant. Discuss any new medication, prescribed or unprescribed, in light of the fact that you are pregnant. This also applies to breastfeeding.

- ***Other drugs*** Keep away from all illegal drugs such as cocaine, marijuana, heroin, LSD and crack, if not for your own sake, then for your baby's.
- ***Eating*** Make sure that you eat a balanced diet, made up mainly of vegetables, fruit, cereals, bread, lean meat, poultry, fish, nuts, milk, cheese, yoghurt and some eggs. Drink eight glasses of water daily. Avoid, or at least limit, sugar, salt, margarine, butter and oil. Keep away from artificially coloured and flavoured foods and those high in preservatives. Do not diet during pregnancy. Talk to your doctor if you are concerned about your weight gain.

You should drink 600 mL of milk, or its calcium equivalent, per day. If you are going to have difficulty taking in enough calcium in this way, talk to your doctor about calcium tablets.

A small amount of tea or coffee is acceptable. Many pregnant women conveniently develop an aversion to tea and coffee.

You may need vitamin and mineral supplements, folic acid and iron supplements. Discuss this with your doctor. Do not assume that because something is labelled 'vitamin', 'herb' or 'natural', that it is harmless. This is definitely not the case. Herbal teas can contain dangerous substances and should be avoided during pregnancy.

- ***Pregnant vegetarians*** Seek professional advice if you want to continue with a vegetarian diet. It will need to be assessed to ensure that it is adequate for you and your baby.
- ***Morning sickness*** The key to relieving pregnancy-based nausea is to have a larger number of small meals. Start the day before you get out of bed with a cup of

SEX DURING PREGNANCY

If you are healthy, you can still enjoy sex during pregnancy. Take care if:

- You have an incompetent cervix. You may have to be stitched and advised to avoid sex
- Bleeding occurs. Consult your doctor immediately
- Your waters have broken
- You have a vaginal or urinary infection
- You have had a previous premature delivery. You may be instructed to avoid orgasm, especially later in the pregnancy

tea and some dry biscuits or toast.

❑ ***Sleep and relaxation*** Ensure that you have regular sleep and relaxation. The hormonal effects in early pregnancy may make you more tired than usual, and in late pregnancy you may be very tired because of the discomfort. Make a regular time to relax during the day, particularly after lunch. Learn some simple relaxation techniques. These will be invaluable, not just during pregnancy, but also during those hectic early baby years.

❑ ***Exercise during pregnancy*** It seems wise to begin a pregnancy fit and healthy. Keep up your level of fitness but you may have to make some concession in the type of exercise you do. Do not begin a strenuous fitness program.

❑ ***Antenatal classes*** These classes provide an opportunity to prepare for what might occur during labour. They also provide a focus for the couple to concentrate on together. Techniques to deal with labour are only guidelines – different techniques will help different couples. Some women find the breathing techniques useful, whereas others do better to follow their natural instincts.

It is important to remember that labour and birth are just a beginning. You will need a lot of energy for the months following. Both parents should be prepared for, and have some understanding of, the demands of parenting.

Is it a boy or a girl?

It is actually the man's semen which will determine the sex of the baby. All female chromosomes are of the X type but sperm can be either X or Y.

If a Y sperm fertilises the egg, it will be a boy.
If an X sperm fertilises the egg the baby will be a girl.

Many people are obsessed with producing a child of one particular sex. Extravagant claims, not supported by scientific proof, are made for various methods which can ensure that this happens. In the long run, a healthy baby, of whatever sex, is what really counts.

CAESARIAN BIRTHS

You may know in advance that you will need a caesarian section if the baby has a very large head, is in a difficult position, or you are unwell. An emergency caesarian may become necessary, because of other factors arising during labour. You may have a 'trial of labour', where if all goes well you will have a vaginal delivery. If not, a caesarian will be performed. It is becoming increasingly popular to have a caesarian under an epidural anaesthetic so you can be aware during the birth

Childbirth

Immense changes have taken place in obstetrics over the last twenty years. The pendulum has swung away from technical intervention and cold hard efficiency towards a more intimate and personal environment. It does seem, however, that all the attention given to seeking out the ultimate childbirth experience seems somewhat misplaced – rather like concentrating only on the wedding and not preparing for the long years of marriage ahead! There are a number of different ways to give birth. Choose one that suits you.

Homebirth or hospital? Homebirth, usually attended by a midwife increases the risk of problems, and should really only be attempted, if at all, by those who are most unlikely to develop any complications. Complications can occur very unexpectedly. The response must be swift and technical facilities readily available. Before you opt for homebirth, discuss all the pros and cons with your doctor.

If you are a private patient in a hospital, you can choose your doctor. Your choice of hospital will be limited to the hospitals your doctor works at. As a public patient or a member of the National Health Service, you can choose any hospital with a maternity section. The doctor or midwives on duty will deliver your baby. If you choose a birthing centre, book early to ensure your place.

Breastfeeding

Many women find breastfeeding easy. However, for some, breastfeeding can be fraught with difficulty and they may need help with technique. Ask the hospital staff or midwife to help you to attach the baby properly to the breast and help you establish breastfeeding. It is no longer fashionable to rub creams into the breasts to prepare them for breastfeeding. Avoid soap, as soap washes away natural secretions that keep nipples supple and more easily able to breastfeed.

Contraception

METHODS OF CONTRACEPTION			
Natural	Mechanical Methods	Surgical Methods	Medical
Natural family planning	IUD or intra-uterine device Condom Diaphragm (cap)	Vasectomy Tubal ligation	Mini-Pill Triphasic and Biphasic Pill Injectable hormones

Oral contraception

The oral contraceptive pill, more commonly called the Pill, is a very effective way of preventing conception. These days there are a number of different types available. The most commonly used is the combined Pill, containing two hormones – an oestrogen and a progesterone. The pills comes in two different packs, a twenty-one-day pack and a twenty-eight-day pack. Both are equally effective, and the only difference is that the twenty-eight-day pack has reminder tablets as well. Some women feel it is easier to take a pill every day rather than having to remember to stop and restart after a week.

How does it work? A simple way of understanding how the Pill works is to consider how successful conception happens. Firstly, an egg must be released, secondly, the sperm must be able to get to the egg to fertilise it and thirdly, the uterus must provide the right environment for the fertilised egg to grow. In fact, the combined contraceptive pill works to make sure that none of these three situations occur, preventing conception.

The Pill does nothing to protect you against sexually transmitted infection. These infections are rife among single, sexually active people in our community. If you are not in a stable, monogamous relationship, you should insist on using condoms to protect yourself.

Triphasic and biphasic pills These are often the first contraceptive pills now prescribed. They are a more recent development of the combined Pill, except that the dosages of oestrogen and progesterone are varied through the month to provide concentrations of hormone closer to the natural levels.

Progestagen-only Pill This type is also known as the mini-Pill. It contains only one type of hormone, a progestagen, and is a lower dose than in the combined Pill. It acts on the cervical mucus, making it thicker and more difficult for sperm to penetrate. Breastfeeding women, women aged over thirty-five, or those who cannot take oestrogen hormones are generally prescribed the mini-Pill. It has a higher failure rate than the other oral contraceptives and can cause irregular bleeding.

Is the Pill effective?

Generally the Pill is very effective but a number of factors can affect how well it functions.

- It is essential that you remember to take it exactly as prescribed. Do not miss taking the Pill.
- The Pill is not effective for about fourteen days. This means that you need to use other methods of contraception for this period. Don't forget that if you change pills, particularly to a lower dose one, you will need extra contraception for the first fourteen days of that cycle.
- Diarrhoea and vomiting can interfere with the Pill's absorption.
- Always discuss with your doctor any other medications you are taking. Some antibiotics prevent the Pill from working.

DO YOU NEED A BREAK?

Women used to be advised to take a break from the Pill every few years as it was thought that continued use without a break was harmful. This is no longer believed to be the case. A break serves no other purpose than to cause an increased rate of unwelcome pregnancies

SIDE EFFECTS OF THE PILL	
Blood clots	The most dangerous side effect of oral contraceptive pills is that they may affect the circulation. Blood clots are a rare complication, but must be watched for
Blood pressure	Some women on the Pill find that their blood pressure rises
Smoking	Women are advised nowadays not to smoke while on the Pill. Smoking is an additional, unnecessary risk for blood pressure, heart disease and stroke
Cervical cancer	The risk of developing this condition is increased a little if you are on the Pill. However, as discussed in the section on cervical cancer, other factors are more important
Liver disorders	Some types of liver disorders are slightly more likely to develop while on the Pill

Side effects do occasionally occur, even with the most recently developed formulations of the Pill. See your doctor – do not suffer in silence

Other forms of contraception

❑ ***Injectable hormones*** In some developed countries, this cannot be promoted as a contraceptive, but in others it is a freely available alternative. Side effects tend to be more pronounced because of the high doses of hormones given.

❑ ***Intra-uterine device (IUD)*** This is a device that is inserted into your uterus by a trained person and left for a number of years. It is thought that the IUD prevents pregnancy by changing the speed at which the egg travels and by making the uterus less hospitable to the egg. It is also probable that the antibodies formed in reaction to the presence of the IUD probably also attack sperm.

The most serious side effect associated with IUD use is the increased chance of developing pelvic infection, possibly resulting in infertility. The chances of developing infection are greater if you have a number of sexual partners. For this reason, the IUD has been used less in single women who have not yet had a family, and is more suited to the married, monogamous woman who has completed or nearly completed her family. The IUD can also cause heavier, more painful periods.

There is a risk of perforating the uterus at the time of insertion. If pregnancy occurs while the IUD is in place, there is an increased chance of it being ectopic, because the IUD does not prevent ectopic pregnancy. The IUD is removed if pregnancy occurs.

❑ ***Condoms*** These are one of the earliest used forms of contraception and are making a comeback. Because of their ability to prevent the spread of infections, such as AIDS, it may be a good idea to use condoms, in all nonmonogamous sexual liaisons. There is a certain community resistance to the use of condoms and considerable public health effort is being directed towards overcoming this resistance.

It is hard to know how effective condoms really are as contraceptives. Some fail because they are of poor quality, others because they are not always used properly. They are more effective if used with spermicidal creams, providing you are not allergic to them.

❑ ***Diaphragms (caps)*** This is a rubber contraceptive device that the woman inserts before intercourse. It forms a barrier, preventing the passage of sperm into the cervical canal. It is more effective if used with spermicidal cream. Effectiveness can be hard to assess because it depends very much on the user's motivation. Diaphragms come in different sizes. A doctor or specially trained nurse will need to fit one for you and show you how to insert it correctly.

❑ ***Natural family planning*** Also known as periodic abstinence, this method works on the theory that if you can successfully identify when a woman is fertile, you can reduce the risk of pregnancy by avoiding sex at that time. There are a number of indicators used to determine the fertile period, including temperature, mucus and calendar methods. Have your doctor explain them to you or attend a course run by Catholic Family Planning Centres who specialise in these methods.

Sterilisation

Many couples are choosing sterilisation as a contraceptive measure once they have completed their families. Before making this choice, it is wise to balance the pros and cons of male sterilisation, called vasectomy, against female sterilisation, called tubal ligation.

- ***Vasectomy*** This operation involves cutting the tube, called the vas deferens, which carries the sperm to the penis. Sperm are still produced, but the body reabsorbs them. Ejaculation (free of sperm) still occurs and sexual drive is not affected. The procedure can be done under a local anaesthetic. A sperm count will need to be done to make sure that the vasectomy has been successful. Vasectomy should be regarded as permanent. Although there have been surgical reversals, this doesn't always work.
- ***Tubal ligation*** There are a number of techniques available, all involving the same basic idea. The tubes are cut, clamped or tied so that fertilisation of the egg cannot occur. You still have normal periods. The operation is usually performed by a gynaecologist and requires a general anaesthetic. It should also be regarded as permanent. Reversals are sometimes attempted with no guarantee of success.

Breastfeeding

Many women regard breastfeeding as an effective contraceptive. It is not. Many women do become pregnant while breastfeeding. All that can be said is that if you compare breastfeeding women (not using contraception), with nonbreastfeeding women (also not using contraception) there will probably be a slightly longer gap between babies in the first group. One problem is that when you are breastfeeding, you just don't know when you are going to have your first ovulation.

Infertility

In many cases of infertility, no specific problem can be found. Continued patience and persistence, adoption or in-vitro fertilisation may provide the solution

Infertility is quite a common problem, affecting ten per cent of couples who try to conceive a child. There are numerous causes. When you stop to consider all the things that have to happen in order to conceive, it is a wonder that fertility occurs as often as it does!

What can be done

A couple should spend a year trying to start a pregnancy before they seek help. After that, it is necessary to undertake a step-by-step investigation of each partner.

Firstly, it is important to obtain a medical history from both partners. Any scrotal or testicular damage, excessive heat or stress in the area, alcohol or smoking, may have affected the man's ability to produce healthy sperm. The best way to check sperm is to do a sperm count and analysis. The man collects this specimen by masturbation for analysis within a few hours.

On the woman's side, it is necessary to know if ovulation is occurring regularly or at all. This can be roughly assessed over a few months, using a temperature chart. Blood tests of hormone levels can confirm the findings. A postcoital (after intercourse) test, which looks at the way in which the sperm are received by the cervical mucus, may also be suggested. Other tests will be suggested according to findings and suspicions at this stage.

There is an increasing incidence to show that pelvic infection in women contributes to the subsequent development of blocked fallopian tubes, and infertility. Tests can check if the woman's tubes are functioning properly. Injections of dye can be used to clear tubes, but more severe blockages will require surgery.

INFECTIONS

Infections, both viral and bacterial, are probably the most frequent cause of illness. These days, the community is most troubled by the apparent increase in sexually transmitted infections, especially AIDS.

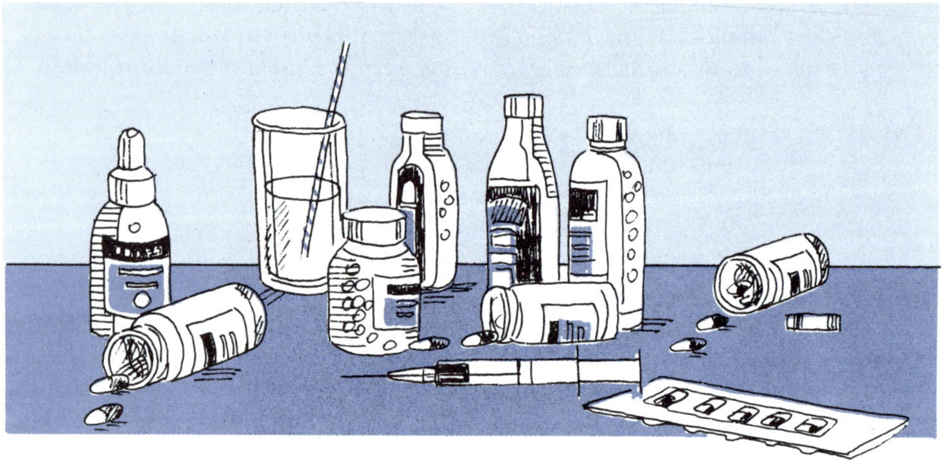

Viral and bacterial infections

Firstly, it is important from a practical point of view, to determine whether an infection is viral or bacterial. If your infection is bacterial you need an antibiotic, if it is viral you do not.

What kinds of infection are caused by bacteria and viruses? Bacterial infections can affect many organs. Commonly occurring bacterial infections cause tonsillitis, pneumonia, middle ear infection, skin infection and sinusitis.

Viral infections can occur in the same parts of the body as bacterial infections. Many commonly occurring and well known illnesses are caused by viruses. Included are the childhood illnesses of measles, mumps, chicken pox and German measles, and others, such as hepatitis A and B, AIDS, glandular fever and influenza.

It is possible to take swabs to identify any bacteria present and assess the most suitable antibiotics. It is usual to initiate treatment without delay. In general, viruses which are smaller organisms cannot be detected directly without blood tests.

Finding a cure Bacteria can live outside cells but viruses can only grow and multiply in living cells. An effective antiviral agent has to kill the virus without killing the cell in which it is living. This makes the search for cures for viral infections a much more difficult exercise.

Tetanus

Tetanus affects any age and can cause death. It occurs mostly in fractured bones where the skin has been broken; penetrating wounds; wounds where a foreign body, such as a wood splinter, soil, dust or horse manure, has penetrated; and injuries in which a lot of soft tissue damage has occurred, such as burns. Tetanus can develop up to three weeks after the injury, but in most cases occurs within seven to ten days.

Childhood tetanus immunisation will protect you for a time but it is wise to keep up your immunity with a single booster injection every ten years. It should include diphtheria vaccine as well. If you sustain an injury that could cause tetanus, you should be vaccinated if it is two or more years since your last booster dose. If it is over ten years since your last booster, you may require two injections. If you do not know whether you have ever completed a full course of immunisation, or more than twenty years have passed since your last tetanus injection, you should have the full course of three injections.

BACTERIAL OR VIRAL?

Bacterial

- Often tonsillitis

Some types of the following

- Pneumonia
- Middle ear infection
- Skin infection
- Sinusitus

Viral

- Measles
- Mumps
- Chickenpox
- German measles
- Hepatitis A and B
- AIDS
- Glandular fever
- Influenza

Genital infections

Monilia

Monilia, also known as Candida albicans and thrush, is a fungus that lives quite normally on our skin, in our mouth, throat, intestines and vagina without causing a problem. It is only if it is allowed to multiply that the symptoms of an infection occur. Monilia infection commonly develops in the vagina of women and the mouths of babies. A course of antibiotics or certain formulations of the contraceptive pill can result in monilial fungal overgrowth and hence infection. In addition, diabetes, drug addiction and certain forms of cancer therapy can result in an increase in this type of vaginal infection.

You may also find that you can develop a monilial infection while pregnant or breastfeeding. However, a large number of women have no idea why they are prone to this infection. We do know that as monilial overgrowth, and hence infection, is favoured by a humid environment, conditions that encourage sweating should be avoided. Therefore, avoid tight jeans and synthetic underwear and pantihose, especially during a flare-up of infection.

Symptoms If you develop a monilial infection, you may notice a thick, white, vaginal discharge and have an itchy vagina. The discomfort of the itch will probably cause you to see your doctor. On examination, the doctor will find a white cheesy substance sticking to the vaginal wall.

If you are a male and you contact genital monilia, (easily caught from a sexual partner and equally easily passed back to her), you too may develop symptoms. The penis may become irritated and red, with some discharge. A number of men with the fungus do not develop symptoms, and so can unknowingly pass it to a sexual partner. For this reason, in recurring attacks of monilia, your doctor may advise both you and your sexual partner to be treated at the same time.

Treatment There are a number of antifungal creams and pessaries on the market. Originally, treatment was for fourteen days. Newer treatments do not have to be used for as long. In addition, tablets can be taken by mouth and there is a new type of tablet reserved for severe recurring conditions. Sexual activity is best avoided. If unavoidable, a condom should be used during treatment. Most women will experience at least one attack of monilia during their lives and, for most, it is easily treated. For an unlucky minority, trying to control recurrent monilia will be a persistent problem. If an underlying reason for recurrent monilia is present, this should be attended to where possible.

Changing the chemical environment of the vagina by wiping the infected area with diluted vinegar (one part vinegar to five parts water) can help to control monilia

Trichomonas

Another common vaginal infection is caused by an organism called trichomonas vaginalis, or trich for short. This infection also causes an itchy discharge. Characteristically, the trichomonas discharge is thin and greenish white with a foul odour. This tends to appear during or just after menstruation. Again men can unknowingly become infected.

Treatment There are a couple of antibiotics generally used to treat this condition. One involves taking four tablets once only. After this, it is important not to have sex or alcohol for forty-eight hours. The other treatment is taken over seven days.

Chlamydia

This organism, also known as chlamydia trachomatis, can cause a variety of human infections. It has recently received much attention because it is a well-known sexually transmitted disease.

Symptoms There may be no indication that you have the infection or, if you are a woman, you can experience vaginal discharge, pelvic pain, menstrual irregularities, inflamed anus (if anal intercourse has taken place), and frequency and burning during urination.

CHLAMYDIA

Doctors are becoming increasingly concerned about a number of features of chlamydia:

- It is a common disease
- It is often a silent disease in that the sufferer may have no symptoms
- Unchecked, it can lead to infertility.
- It is easily spread and increasing

Symptoms in men may include burning and frequency during urination and prostate or anal inflammation. Your doctor can diagnose the infection in the absence of symptoms with special pathology tests. If you are in any doubt, discuss these tests with your doctor.

The danger of chlamydia in women is that it can spread from the vagina to the tubes and uterus, causing infertility, ectopic pregnancy or a genital abscess. In men, the infection can spread to the prostate, also resulting in infertility. Babies who pass through an infected birth canal can also become infected, developing eye and lung diseases.

Who is at risk? The people at risk are those who have had more than one sexual partner fairly recently, or any new sexual relationship with someone who has had other sexual partners.

It is worth remembering that condoms provide some protection against the transmission of chlamydia infection and other sexually transmitted diseases.

Treatment Fortunately, chlamydia can be eradicated with appropriate antibiotics. It is essential that all sexual partners of both involved partners are also treated. It is important to diagnose the chlamydia infection before complications arise.

Genital Warts

There are a number of different wart viruses. In general, only the genital type virus infects the genital area. A number of studies point to an association between certain genital warts and genital cancer. It often takes about four to six weeks for warts to appear after the infection. However, there are exceptions. Sometimes the wart virus may not present itself until long after the initial contact. If you have had a number of sexual partners, it can be difficult to work out the source of infection. To further complicate the issue, a number of people infected with the wart virus will have no indication of its presence. Not all cases of genital warts seem to be accounted for by sexual transmission.

Treatment There are a number of treatments available. A special wart paint containing podophyllin can be applied every week. It should not be given to pregnant women. Great care needs to be exercised in ensuring that only the warts are treated. For this reason, it is generally advised that your doctor applies the paint. The warts can be frozen or burnt off.

Genital herpes is caused by a similar virus to the one which causes the more familiar herpes, commonly known as cold sores

Genital Herpes

The herpes virus can also cause a sexually transmitted infection. Genital herpes is fairly common, affecting up to fifteen per cent of women of childbearing age. It is often a recurrent disease, although recurring attacks tend to be milder. The very first attack of herpes is usually the most severe.

Symptoms Herpes infection produces painful blisters which eventually burst, crust and dry up. Pain is the main problem experienced by the sufferer. Intercourse is painful and should be avoided so as not to spread the virus.

Treatment Traditionally, treatment has included rest, daily salt bathing, urinating in the bath (when urination is painful), and local anaesthetic creams. There is a relatively new drug available which has a place in the treatment of some genital herpes infections, particularly the recurrent severe type.

Recurrent herpes is more likely to occur if you are run down. Keeping up a healthy lifestyle, without drugs and alcohol, getting enough sleep and avoiding stress may lessen the chance of a recurrence.

Herpes and pregnancy It is important that a pregnant woman informs her treating doctor if either she or her husband have had genital herpes. A baby born through a herpes-infected birth canal can become seriously ill. Your obstetrician will advise whether a vaginal delivery is possible.

HIV infection and AIDS

Human immunodeficiency virus infection can progress from one stage to another, the most serious stage being AIDS (acquired immunodeficiency syndrome).

Who is at risk? Transmission of the AIDS or HIV virus can occur during sexual activity. Certain types of sexual activity are more likely to result in infection, for example, anal intercourse. For this reason, the homosexual community is at great risk from AIDS.

Sharing of needles (often practised by intravenous drug abusers) and blood and blood product transfusion, have also been associated with infection. Modern methods of screening blood have reduced the incidence of this latter case. We also know that an infected mother can pass the infection to her child in the womb. There are also a few reports of infection acquired from breastfeeding.

HIV infection The usual stages of HIV infection are described in the following table, but not everybody infected will progress in this way. Some remain antibody positive without symptoms and so are still at risk of passing the illness to others. At present, there is neither an effective treatment to halt the progression of the disease – or a vaccine to immunise against it, as there is with the more common disease of hepatitis B.

At present there is no cure for AIDS. Management of the disease is directed towards community education about prevention and safe sex practices

STAGES OF HIV INFECTION	
Stage 1	Acute infection with many flu-like symptoms
Stage 2	Apparent recovery with no symptoms
Stage 3	Characterised by persistent enlargement of the lymph nodes
Stage 4	Full-blown AIDS or AIDS-related complex (ARC) with a long list of possible symptoms and intercurrent illnesses At this stage, the body's ability to fight infection has lessened and continues to fall dramatically The patient becomes ridden with infections that an increasingly weak body is unable to fight off Death eventually follows

How to avoid the disease Avoiding infection means avoiding high-risk situations, such as the sharing of needles and unprotected sex outside an exclusively monogamous relationship. Unprotected sexual intercourse with a new partner whose previous sexual behaviour is not fully known carries great danger. In this situation it is always wise to adopt safe sex practices.

In addition, if there is a possibility that you may have acquired a sexually transmitted disease, contact your doctor immediately. Unchecked sexually transmitted diseases can lead to devastating consequences.

WHAT IS SAFE SEX?

- Safest: mutual masturbation, vaginal intercourse with condom (no breakage), dry kissing
- Less safe: wet kissing, oral sex where secretions and ejaculate are not swallowed, anal intercourse with a condom
- Least safe: anal sex without condoms, vaginal sex without condoms, receptive oral intercourse and shared sex toys

Hepatitis B

Hepatitis B is an infectious, potentially fatal disease of the liver which is increasing. It can also result in the development of liver cirrhosis or liver cancer later in life in about twenty per cent of carriers.

Symptoms A person who has hepatitis B can present in a number of ways. Firstly, they may become very ill with symptoms that include fever, vomiting, jaundice (yellowing of skin and eyes) and tiredness. Some people develop the infection without realising. It may only come to their attention if blood tests show that they have had hepatitis B some time in the past. After an initial attack of hepatitis B, some people become immune, and won't pass on the infection. Others become carriers and can go on passing the illness to other people.

Who is at risk?

Others who are possibly at risk are young children who attend child-care situations and associate with children in the high-risk categories, those who accidentally acquire the infection by stepping on a used syringe, or by accidental cross-infection with others during dental procedures. Many doctors argue that, at present, the risk to those people not in high-risk groups is small.

At present, migrants and visitors from countries where the disease is rife are not being screened, yet we know that the carrier rate of this disease is increasing. We may need to adopt a more aggressive approach to restrict the spread of the disease.

HEPATITIS A

- More common than hepatitis B
- Primarily affects children and young adults
- Usually spread via contaminated food
- It can spread rapidly through a community

HEPATITIS B HIGH RISK GROUPS

- intravenous drug users
- male homosexuals
- both heterosexuals and bisexuals who have a number of sexual partners
- people in institutions and those looking after them
- health care workers who have contact with blood or body fluids
- certain racial groups
- family members of hepatitis B carriers
- family members of acute hepatitis B patients
- babies whose mothers are carriers of hepatitis B
- patients receiving blood products (for example those with haemophilia)

How does the disease spread? The hepatitis B virus lives in all body fluids, including sweat, tears, saliva, vaginal secretions and semen. The infection may therefore be transmitted by sexual intercourse, use of an infected needle, razor blade, toothbrush or by being bitten by a carrier.

Can hepatitis be prevented? There is a vaccine available that can reduce the risk of getting the disease. It is not a cure and must be given before you have contracted the infection. Vaccination involves a course of three injections. The first two are generally given at least one month apart and the next, at least five to six months later. The vaccine should be given to people in high-risk categories but, at present, the cost is limiting its use. Check with your doctor if you think you may be a candidate for the vaccine. The course of vaccination can be followed up with a blood test to establish if you have developed immunity. For those who have not, a fourth injection may be advised. Just how long immunity lasts is not known. One booster injection may be required every three to five years.

Urinary infections

Urinary infections, such as cystitis (inflammation of the bladder) and urethritis (inflammation of the urethra), occur more often in women than men. These infections, singly or in combination, constitute a lower urinary tract infection (UTI).

Cystitis is a very common condition, affecting most women at least once in their lifetime and some unfortunate women, many times.

Who is at risk?

There are clear physiological reasons why women are more susceptible to urinary tract infections than men are. Usually, the source of the infection is from outside the body. Because women have shorter urethras with openings closer to the anal opening, bacteria have a shorter distance to travel to infect the female urinary tract. Often these bacteria are harmless in their normal environment in the intestine, but multiply in the lower urinary tract resulting in the symptoms of infection. Vigorous sexual activity can also inflame a woman's urethra and introduce bacteria into the urinary tract. Some women are able to control the sexually related urinary symptoms by regularly emptying their bladder before and after sex or by using an antiseptic or antibiotic cream before sex.

The urethra is responsible for carrying infection to the bladder and urine away from it. In males, it is a tube about 20 cm long, running from the bladder to the penis. In women, the urethra is only about 4 cm long

Symptoms Most commonly, there is an unpleasant burning sensation when urinating, along with the need to urinate frequently but passing only small amounts. Sometimes there is blood in the urine. At this point, you can help yourself by drinking lots of clear fluids (for example, water) to maintain your urine flow. This can help flush away the infection. Unfortunately, you may be tempted not to take fluids so as to avoid the unpleasant sensation of passing urine, but you should persevere. If you are suffering these symptoms, you should visit your doctor as treatment is available to reduce your symptoms.

Treatment Your doctor may suggest a mid-stream urine specimen for pathology testing to identify the particular bacterium, which is causing the infection. Urine is collected by urinating a little into the toilet bowl and then catching a small amount of the mid-flow of urine in a sterile container. The remaining urine is then passed directly into the toilet bowl. The reason for collecting the urine in this way is that the first part of the urine flow is most likely to be contaminated with bacteria from the outside of the urinary opening.

It is usual to prescribe an antibiotic after collecting the specimen, even before the test results are known. If an infection is found, a second urine sample, called a follow-up, is taken after treatment to check that all traces of the infection have disappeared. Sometimes women can develop recurrent bouts of urinary infection. If you suffer recurrent infections it is certainly worth trying to empty your bladder before and after sex to see if this has any effect. Remember, always wipe or wash from the front to the back (i.e. urethra to vagina to anus) – never in the reverse direction as this can cause infection.

It is possible for urinary infection to ascend to the kidneys. The patient is usually sick with high fever, chills and back pain. Immediate medical attention should be sought. Keeping up your fluid intake is a wise precaution.

Urinary infection in children

Any child who is unwell for no apparent cause may have a urinary tract infection. This can also be true in the elderly. It is important that urinary infection in children is properly treated and followed up. Your doctor needs to exclude any developmental abnormality that could lead to serious kidney disease.

SERIOUS DISEASES

Many serious diseases are affected by the pressures and stresses of today's busy lifestyle. Taking steps to reduce stress and paying attention to diet and exercise can play a preventive role.

Heart disease and strokes

There are certain risk factors that increase your chances of having a heart attack. The more of them you have, the more likely you are to suffer a heart attack. However, we all know people who defy statistics. They smoke, eat the wrong foods, never exercise and they don't have heart attacks. Many people find this hard to understand. An analogy may help: you can take precautions to cross a road at a pedestrian crossing, or you can ignore all precautions and cross the road just beyond a blind curve. Your chances of being hit by a car are higher in the latter case but it is not inconceivable that you may be hit on the pedestrian crossing. So it is with risk factors for a particular disease. You can minimise the risks by obeying health guidelines or you can increase your risk by living a more dangerous lifestyle.

Not all risk factors can be decreased. Some, such as heredity, are beyond your control. Others, such as smoking and diet, are well within your control. At the present, passive smoking (i.e. inhaling the cigarette smoke of others) is outside your control but future legislation may change that.

You can reduce your risk of heart attack by reducing your level of cholesterol and blood fats and giving up smoking. Have your cholsterol tested by your doctor. If it is high, you will need to modify your diet and then be retested. If it still remains high, you may need prescribed drugs. As for smoking, it is one of the greatest contributory causes of heart disease, not to mention cancer and other ailments. Stop smoking!

High blood pressure

Many lifestyle factors contribute to high blood pressure and there is a lot you can do to protect yourself. (See table below)

If lifestyle measures are not successful, medication is often required. Once you are prescribed medication, it is usual for your doctor to check your blood pressure regularly to see if you require a change in prescription.

HOW TO LOWER YOUR BLOOD PRESSURE

- Lose weight
- Stop smoking
- Drink less alcohol
- Exercise regularly
- Use less salt

Cancer

There are many factors that seem to be associated with the different types of cancer. Some of these are:

Smoking Smoking is linked to many different types of cancer as well as lung cancer.

Food There is much research into the association between particular foodstuffs and particular cancers. So far, there have not been enough answers to give very specific advice, but some general points have emerged.

- The cruciferous vegetables such as cabbage, broccoli, Brussel sprouts and cauliflower may help reduce bowel cancer
- A high intake of salt-cured and pickled foods have been linked with stomach cancer
- High fat intake is also linked with some cancers

Generally, we should all eat a healthy balanced diet with high fibre grains and fruits and vegetables as outlined in Health and Diet on p 4.

Family history We do know that certain cancers, including breast and bowel cancer, tend to run in families. Tests exist to detect both of these cancers early. Self-examination and regular examination by your doctor will help detect breast cancer in the early stages. Special X-rays, called mammograms, are also helpful in identifying early changes in breasts.

Screening for bowel cancer involves checking the stool for blood and passing a tube into the bowel so that any suspicious lesions can be viewed and biopsied if necessary. Alternatively, a barium enema, a special type of X-ray in which the barium is used to coat the walls of the bowel, may be used.

Sick-building syndrome

There are many symptoms being seen in some workers in modern office buildings. Those who get the symptoms work in air-conditioned buildings without windows that can be opened. Symptoms include headache; lack of energy; stuffy nose; dry throat; sore or dry eyes; nausea; dry itchy skin and dizziness. The problem might affect up to a third of modern office buildings, and about 10 to 30 per cent of the occupants. Causes are not yet known, but there may be many things that contribute, such as overheating and lack of ventilation. Recently workers have been advised to bring plants to work. Apparently they can make the office environment healthier.

Diabetes

Diabetes refers to a condition in which the body does not handle sugar properly. A high blood sugar level results, and sugar appears in the urine. This can be detected by a simple blood test. Diabetes can have many complications involving the heart, eyes, skin, kidney and circulation. There are two types of diabetes. (See table) Type 1 (insulin dependent) occurs in children and young adults. Its onset is often dramatic with noticeable symptoms including changed thirst, tiredness, weight loss and a craving for sugar. Because the body is producing no insulin, the substance which promotes sugar absorption in the blood, insulin injections are required to control the diabetes. Type 2 (non insulin dependent) occurs in older adults (the cut-off point between the two is generally age forty). Type 2 is often a more insidious condition. It may only be picked up on a routine urine or blood test. It tends to run in families, and can often be treated by modifying diet. In addition, blood sugar lowering tablets or insulin may need to be prescribed.

OCCURRENCE		SYMPTOMS	CONTROL
Type 1 Diabetes	Children and young adults	Thirst, tiredness, weight loss, sugar craving	Insulin injections
Type 2 Diabetes	Older adults	Thirst, obesity, excessive food intake, infection, high urine output	Diet modification, blood sugar lowering tablets

Chronic fatigue syndrome

This disease was formerly known as myalgic encephalomyelitis and is commonly named by the media as 'the yuppie flu'. At present it remains a mystery disease, affecting mainly, but not only, young female adults. Some doctors believe that it occurs following a viral infection. Others argue that this is not always the case. Still others that it is not a disease at all!

The term chronic fatigue refers to the main symptoms of extreme tiredness for no readily apparent reason. The use of the word encephalomyelitis derives from the other common symptoms of headache and pain. Inability to concentrate, memory problems and mood changes may also develop. Physical effort worsens the feelings of tiredness.

The diagnosis should only apply if the following situations occur: fatigue and other documented symptoms with no response to rest, for at least six months in spite of a 50 per cent reduction in daily activity and other diagnoses (including infection, hormonal abnormalities, psychiatric disease and cancer) have been excluded.

Many people are given an incorrect diagnosis if the medical criteria have not been adhered to. At present, the cause of the disease is not known.

Legionnaire's disease

This was first recognised in 1977, following an epidemic of the disease among US war veterans attending a Philadelphia Legionnaire's conference. Ten per cent of those attending the conference became ill, sparking off investigations which led to the discovery of the bacteria responsible for the disease.

The disease has probably been around (but unrecognised) as a form of pneumonia for years. It is known that the bacteria responsible for Legionnaire's disease like to live in water, and can be found in contaminated air conditioners, vaporisers and water heaters.

The elderly, chronically ill and smokers are more likely to be affected. As the illness is caused by a bacterium, taking the correct antibiotics can cure it. No vaccine to prevent the condition exists.

YOUR A to Z

A

Acne
Chapter 3
The term acne can cover pimples, blackheads, whiteheads, cysts and swellings, caused by a blockage to the oil glands on the skin. Many frightening myths abound about acne. There are a number of simple treatments available or certain antibiotics can be prescribed by the doctor. The usual way to control acne is in a step-wise manner proceeding from the simplest methods of control to the most complicated.

Alcohol
Chapter 1
Alcohol damages many parts of the body including the brain, liver and kidneys. It is associated with road accidents, marital and family distress, violent crime and employment problems.

Allergies
Chapter 4
These are a series of chemical responses by the body to rid it of an offending agent or allergen, e.g. grass, dust, pollen. Asthma and eczema may develop as part of an allergic response. Asthma is often seen in members of the same family.

Desensitising injections work well for seasonal grass and pollen allergy whereas medications (such as antihistamines and nasal sprays) can also be given for the treatment of allergies.

Amniocentesis
Chapter 7
A test, usually reserved for pregnant women over the age of thirty-five years, which detects Down's syndrome and other abnormalities in the fetus. It also detects the sex of the child.

Animal bites
Chapter 2
Bites or stings from nonpoisonous or uninfected animals require cooling and antiseptic cream. Bites from poisonous creatures need immediate action from a doctor or hospital, especially if swelling around the throat and face result in breathing problems.

People who are allergic to stings need fast action with emergency medical treatment. Pressure immobilisation (a technique of bandaging) prevents poisons circulating widely through the bloodstream.

Anorexia nervosa
Chapter 1
A life threatening condition which starts with a desire to lose weight by strictly controlling food intake. The sufferer becomes extremely thin and may also experience episodes of overeating and self-induced vomiting.

Antibiotics
Chapter 2
The large number of antibiotics on the market are used to treat bacterial infection only. Commonly used antibiotics include penicillin, erythromycin, sulphonamides and tetracyclines. Different organisms respond to different antibiotics. Sometimes a sample from the infected area may be sent to the

laboratory for analysis to identify the organism.

Antidiarrhoea medicines
Chapter 4
It is advisable not to use over-the-counter medications when treating diarrhoea, particularly in children. Treat by diet with plenty of clear fluids and only dry biscuits, rice, toast and honey. Fatty foods, dairy foods and vegetables should be avoided and a doctor consulted if symptoms persist.

Antihistamines
Chapter 2
There are a large number of these preparations on the market. They are used to treat allergies and hay fever. Drowsiness can be a side effect associated with their use.

Antihypertensives
Chapter 2
This is the name given to the large and diverse collection of drugs available on prescription to lower blood pressure. Prescribing for blood pressure can be a very individualised process. Each drug has a number of precautions associated with its use.

Anti-inflammatory drugs
Chapter 2
These drugs are prescribed to alleviate joint inflammation associated with muscle, tendon or joint injury. All drugs in this group have the ability to cause irritation of the stomach lining.

Aspirin and paracetamol
Chapter 2
Although aspirin can be used to relieve minor pains and fevers, it is best to avoid its use in children and teenagers. Paracetamol-containing mixtures are best for children and teenagers.

Asthma
Chapter 4
This may also be termed allergic, wheezy or asthmatic bronchitis. It commonly occurs at all ages. Children have a good chance of growing out of it. The wheezing sound is caused when the air passes through the narrowed, swollen airway. Exercise, allergies, infections, weather changes and stress can provoke attacks. Medications prescribed by your doctor are available for treatment.

Astigmatism
Chapter 3
This is a problem in which the cornea varies in curvature. It can occur with short or long-sightedness or by itself. Treatment is by the use of corrective glasses.

B

Back problems
Chapter 3
Low back pain causes much suffering and pain to many people. By following simple rules to care for your back, recurrent pain can be prevented. It is crucial that muscles are exercised and strengthened. Medication such as anti-inflammatory drugs may be prescribed. Hospitalisation, traction and surgery may be needed for severe cases.

Bacterial and viral infections
Chapter 8
Bacterial infections can be determined by taking swabs and culturing them in a laboratory. After identification of the bacteria, the most suitable antibiotic can be prescribed. Viruses are smaller organisms and require blood tests to detect their presence (the immune response of the body to the viral infection can be measured). Common bacterial infections include tonsillitis, pneumonia, ear and skin infections. Common viral infections include the childhood illnesses of measles, mumps, chicken pox and influenza.

Barium meal or enema
Chapter 1
This is a special X-ray designed to study the bowel. The barium coats the bowel so the X-rays can pick up the outline. Polyps and tumours can be identified this way.

Blocked nose
Chapter 4
Over-enthusiastic use of nose drops for children can cause problems. It is better to humidify the air for a while before resorting to paediatric strength nose drops.

Blood tests
Chapter 1
There are many different types of blood tests required for different purposes. Blood grouping is required before major surgery and during pregnancy.

Body contouring or sculpting
Chapter 3
This is the use of plastic surgery to

reshape many different parts of the body. It is not an alternative to losing weight.

Breastfeeding
Chapter 7
For many women, breastfeeding works well. For others it can be fraught with difficulty. Breastfeeding and bottle feeding both have advantages and disadvantages, and much depends on the needs and preferences of both mother and child.

Breast reduction, lifts, enlargement, reconstruction
Chapter 3
This surgery can reshape and reposition the breasts as well as remove tissue to make the breasts smaller. A prosthesis inserted into the breasts can make them larger. It is possible to reconstruct a breast after mastectomy.

Broken bones
Chapter 2
If it is suspected that a bone has been broken then an X-ray will be performed. A cast is applied to keep bone fragments in position. Sometimes fractured bones require the use of pins and plates to hold them together.

Bronchoscopy
Chapter 1
This involves passing an instrument through the mouth or nose to view the lining of the air passages. Specimens can be obtained for diagnosis and treatment of cancer and infection.

Bulimia nervosa
Chapter 1
This condition is characterised by the consumption of huge amounts of food followed by self-induced vomiting or laxative use.

Bunions
Chapter 3
The big toe points to the side. Women usually develop this condition. Squashing feet into ill-fitting/high-heeled shoes can make it worse. Surgery is a final option.

Burns
Chapter 2
Immediate treatment is the application of cold water (not ice) to the affected area for 10 to 30 minutes. Pain relief needs to be adequate, and strict asepsis must be maintained, as infection can develop in burn areas. See a doctor or hospital casualty department to assess the burn.

C

Caesarian birth
Chapter 7
This method of giving birth involves delivery of the baby through an abdominal incision, under an epidural or general anaesthetic. An emergency caesarian may become necessary if certain factors arise during labour, or if the baby has a big head or is in a difficult position.

Callus
Chapter 3
This develops in an area constantly being rubbed by ill-fitting or high-heeled shoes. Calluses are not generally painful and can be removed by a chiropodist (podiatrist) if necessary.

Cancer and food
Chapter 1
A lot of research continues to try to associate particular foodstuffs with particular cancers. Cabbages and cauliflowers it is believed may help reduce the onset of bowel cancer, whereas salt-cured and pickled foods have been linked with stomach cancer. General advice involves eating a healthy balanced diet.

Cancer, cervical
Chapter 5
This is one of the biggest killers of women over the age of forty years in developed countries. The cervical/PAP smear test detects pre-cancerous changes in the cervix and cervical cancer in women. It is essential that all women have a smear test at least every three years, if not every year, and every three to five years after a hysterectomy. The pre-cancerous changes are treatable, preventing invasive cancer.

Cancer, detection of
Chapter 5
Some cancers tend to run in family groups, especially breast and bowel cancers. It is wise to have regular checks and undergo screening tests as advised by your own doctor.

Cataracts
Chapter 3
A cloudiness or thickening in the lens of the eye is called a cataract. These most commonly occur with age. Once a cataract is dense it

may be removed. The faulty lens is replaced with glasses, contact lenses or a plastic lens implant.

CAT scan
Chapter 1
This new type of X-ray first developed for evaluating the brain is now used for the rest of the body as well. It gives a picture of the organ being studied.

Chest X-ray
Chapter 1
This provides information about the lungs, heart, major blood vessels and surrounding bony cage. A chest X-ray may be ordered if an infection, cancer or any other lung disease is suspected.

Chicken pox
Chapter 1
This itchy rash is a very infectious viral disease, commonly occurring between the ages of two and eight years. It is no longer contagious after the skin lesions have dried. Antihistamines and lotions can be applied to the rash and paracetamol given for fever and discomfort.

Childbirth
Chapter 7
There are many ways in which birth can take place. Investigate all the options and discuss the pros and cons with your doctor before a decision is reached.

Chlamydia
Chapter 8
This organism, chlamydia trachomatis, causes a variety of human infections and is a well known sexually transmitted disease. The sufferer may experience either no symptoms or a number of symptoms including vaginal discharge, pelvic pain and menstrual irregularities in women. It can cause infertility, ectopic pregnancy or a genital abscess. Treatment for both partners is with appropriate antibiotics.

Chorionic villus biopsy
Chapter 7
This test, eight to ten weeks into pregnancy, detects Down's Syndrome or other chromosomal abnormalities in the fetus. It is usually carried out on women over the age of thirty-five when the risks of fetal abnormality are greatly increased.

Chronic fatigue syndrome (myalgic encephalomyelitis)
Chapter 9
Named by the media as 'yuppie flu', this remains a mystery disease. Its main symptoms are extreme tiredness and exhaustion, often accompanied by headache and pain. Self-help groups are available to give support. Research is investigating an immune basis to the disease, with treatments being tested to help sufferers.

Circumcision
Chapter 4
Current medical opinion sees no health benefit in excision of the foreskin, and circumcision is no longer routinely carried out. However, if for any reason it is carried out, then it is safer after the newborn period. Attention to cleanliness should keep the uncircumcised penis clean and free from infection.

Colic
Chapter 4
Colic, often blamed for babies crying is not due to bad parenting. Calm reassurance is probably the best management approach.

Continuous ECG
Chapter 1
A 24-hour Holter monitor provides a continuous ECG recording over twenty-four hours. This test may need to be repeated over a few days to provide useful information.

Contraception
Chapter 7
There are many different ways to prevent contraception, the most common being the use of the contraceptive Pill.

Other methods include the use of a condom, the intrauterine device (IUD), diaphragms (caps), injectable hormones, by sterilisation and natural family planning. Some couples use a combination of methods.

Cortisone creams
Chapter 2
These creams, prescribed for skin lesions, should be treated with respect and used for short periods of time and only in the situation for which they were originally prescribed.

Cough mixtures
Chapter 2
Expectorants aim to liquefy the mucus of a productive cough, making it easier to expel. Warm drinks and inhalations are also helpful.

Cough suppressants reduce the desire to cough in a non-productive cough.

Croup and coughing spasm
Chapter 4
These are often best treated with humidification. This can be achieved by steaming up the bathroom or investing in or hiring a humidifier.

Cuts
Chapter 2
All cuts and wounds other than those only affecting the skin and underlying fatty tissue require medical assessment. Immediate treatment for trivial wounds is to clean well with soap and water and apply antiseptic. A tetanus injection may be required.

Cystoscopy
Chapter 1
This test involves passing a tube through the urethra into the bladder in order to view the bladder directly. Sometimes dye is introduced followed by X-rays.

D

Dermabrasions and chemical face-peel
Chapter 3
Mechanical dermabrasion uses an instrument that effectively sands off the outer layer of the skin. The skin heals and is tighter. Chemical face-peel uses a mixture that burns off the skin in a controlled way. Olive and dark skin does not respond well to this treatment.

Dermatitis and eczema
Chapter 3
Dermatitis is an inflammation of the skin. There are many types of dermatitis including seborrhoeic and contact dermatitis and neurodermatitis.

Eczema may develop in childhood and tends to run in families. Treatment is available for these conditions. Consult your own doctor for advice.

Diabetes
Chapter 9
This is a condition in which a high blood sugar level results from the inability of the body to absorb sugar properly. *Type 1* occurs in children and young adults. Insulin injections are required to control the diabetes. *Type 2* occurs in older adults and is fairly common. It can often be treated by modifying diet. Diabetes can result in many complications such as heart disease, eye, skin, kidney and circulation problems.

Diarrhoea and vomiting
Chapter 4
An adequate intake of fluids is important to prevent dehydration during a period of vomiting or diarrhoea, particularly in children. It is essential to eliminate dairy and fatty foods, as well as most fresh fruit and vegetables in the recovery phase.

E

Ears, foreign bodies in
Chapter 3
Syringing is usually inadvisable and the inserted material is better removed under direct visualisation by a skilled person.

Ear wax
Chapter 3
The function of ear wax is to trap particles of dust and dirt and transport them to the body exterior. This is quite an efficient cleaning system. Do not probe the ear with cotton wool buds or match sticks, as only the outer shell of the ear needs cleaning with a damp cloth.

Electrocardiogram (ECG)
Chapter 1
This test detects irregular heart beats by giving off a distinctive wave form for each beat. An ECG tracing also shows damage to the heart muscle.

Endoscopy, gastroscopy and colonoscopy
Chapter 1
These three investigations use the same principle. A tube is passed into a particular part of the gastrointestinal tract under anaesthesia. This allows the doctor direct visualisation as well as the opportunity to sample and photograph the areas of gut.

Erythema infectiosum
(slapped face syndrome)
Chapter 4
This condition is characterised by distinctive red cheeks, with the rash lasting a few days. It may be accompanied by fever, loss of appetite and sore joints.

Exercise
Chapter 1
If you are planning an exercise program, discuss your plans with

a doctor. The current interest in exercise is a positive and healthy trend as long as common sense and moderation are used. Do not do too much too soon.

Exercise or stress ECG
Chapter 1
This type of ECG records stress on the heart during exercise. This testing requires close supervision.

F

Face lift (rhytidectomy)
Chapter 3
This is a surgical technique that raises the facial skin to remove folds and lines. A face-lift will not create beauty where it was not present before and will last only eight to ten years. Complications can occur.

Fever
Chapter 4
In children, fever is lowered by giving plenty of fluids, paracetamol mixture and by sponging or bathing with tepid water.

Fibre
Chapter 1
The benefits of a diet, rich in fibre are now well recognised in the community. A high fibre diet encourages normal bowel function and may prevent a number of diseases, including bowel cancer.

G

Gastroenteritis, acute
Chapter 4
The onset of this infection in children is often sudden and accompanied by vomiting, diarrhoea and fever, with dehydration in severe cases. Prevent dehydration by giving adequate fluids such as special oral rehydration solutions. Fatty and dairy foods, vegetables and fruit should be avoided. Severe acute gastroenteritis may require hospital admission for the administration of intravenous fluids.

Genital herpes
Chapter 8
This is a common, recurring disease, the first attack being the most severe. The disease presents as a group of blisters that burst, crust and dry up. Treatment involves rest, bathing with salt, and local anaesthetic creams. A new drug exists for severe or recurrent infections. Genital herpes is a very infectious sexually transmitted disease.

Genital warts
Chapter 8
Warts appear four to six weeks, or longer, after the initial infection. Treatment includes a special wart paint but it is not to be used by pregnant women. It is essential that the paint be only applied to the warts. A doctor should apply this treatment.

German measles (rubella)
Chapter 4
Sometimes noticeable symptoms such as a fever, swollen lymph glands and a rash can occur. German measles can cause disastrous effects to an unborn baby if a pregnant woman becomes infected. It is aimed to vaccinate all children to eradicate the disease.

Glandular fever
Chapter 4
This viral infection occurs most commonly in adolescents and young adults. Diagnosis and treatment, comprising adequate rest, fluids and paracetamol for fever and pain are needed.

Glaucoma
Chapter 3
There are different types of glaucoma. It can result in a loss of vision. It is important to have regular checks by a specialist eye doctor (opthalmologist). Daily eye drops are prescribed and pills may be given as well.

Glue ears (serous or secretory otitis media)
Chapter 3
This condition develops when a thick, sticky uninfected fluid develops behind the ear drum. There are no symptoms except for an occasional deafness. Sometimes long-term medications are taken, but surgery to insert grommets (ventilation tubes) is sometimes necessary.

Growing pains
Chapter 4
This name is often given to pains in young children which have no

explanation. They often respond to paracetamol and reassurance.

H

Headaches
Chapter 2
A headache is rarely due to serious and dangerous causes, but if you are worried, or have a new type of headache, seek a medical opinion. Tension headaches are common and due to spasm in the muscles of the neck and head. Headaches can be caused by high blood pressure, meningitis and encephalitis, brain tumours and bleeding in the brain area.

Head injury
Chapter 2
Observe a person with a head injury for at least forty-eight hours after the injury, as head injuries can cause serious illness. Changes in behaviour such as excessive sleepiness, persistent headache, vomiting and the appearance of unequal pupils, require immediate consultation with a doctor.

Hepatitis B
Chapter 8
This often silent disease of the liver can cause liver cirrhosis or liver cancer and even death. It can also be passed to others. Some people show symptoms such as fever, vomiting, jaundice (yellowing of the skin and eyes) and tiredness. Hepatitis B is known to live in all body fluids. There is a vaccine available that reduces chances of getting the disease.

Herbs
Chapter 1
Care should be taken with herbal remedies and they should never be given to children and babies. A number are known to be toxic or there may be contamination present from other ingredients.

HIV infection
Chapter 8
Human immunodeficiency virus (HIV) can take various forms which progress from one stage to another, the most serious condition being AIDS. Transmission occurs mostly through certain types of sexual activity, sharing of needles by intravenous drug abusers, and by blood and blood product transfusion. Safe sexual practices and avoiding the other risk factors can prevent infection.

Hormone replacement therapy (HRT)
Chapter 5
The two different types of hormone given are oestrogen, usually given alone to women who have had hysterectomies, and a combination of oestrogen and progesterone for those women who still have a womb. Consult a doctor sometime before menopause if you are contemplating hormone replacement therapy.

Hyperactivity
Chapter 4
A term that is often used indiscriminately, to describe certain behaviour patterns in children. Diet management, drugs, psychiatric and psychosocial modification are all helpful in dealing with behavioural problems in children.

Hysterectomy
Chapter 5
This is the surgical removal of a woman's womb. This may be due to a physical disease such as fibroids, pelvic infection or cancer. In salpingo-oophorectomy the tubes and ovaries are also removed.

I

Impotence
Chapter 6
Psychological and/or physical reasons can contribute to the inability of a man to maintain an erection in order to have sexual intercourse. Physical treatments are available as well as general counselling to lower anxieties and increase sexual responsiveness.

Incontinence
Chapter 5
Inability to control the evacuation of urine (or faeces). A number of types can occur including stress incontinence (after coughing, sneezing, exercising), dribble incontinence (leakage occurs without provocation), overflow, urge and flooding incontinence.

Infertility
Chapter 7
This is a common problem affecting ten per cent of couples. A step-by-step investigation is undertaken of both partners. It is usually suggested that you try to conceive for about a year before you seek help. Often no problems can be found.

L

Legionnaire's disease
Chapter 9
The bacterium causing this disease lives in water and has been found in contaminated air conditioners, vaporisers and water heaters. It is possible to cure the disease with the correct antibiotics.

Low blood sugar (hypoglycaemia)
Chapter 1
This is a rare medical condition which is frequently diagnosed inappropriately by nonmedical personnel. Diabetes is the opposite of high blood sugar.

M

Masturbation
Chapter 6
Current opinion holds that masturbation is a healthy, normal sexual outlet. Teach children that although it is acceptable, it is private, and not to be practised in front of others.

Medical check-up
Chapter 1
Each adult should be checked for blood pressure, cholesterol, blood fats, urine and weight. Adult women need regular breast checks, cervical/PAP smear tests and pelvic examinations. A full personal and family medical history provides the doctor with the information needed to advise you on the need and frequency for other tests.

Medication - how to take
Chapter 2
Medicines should be taken only as prescribed. Antibiotic medications require the full course to be taken irrespective of when symptoms cease. Other medication may only be used as long as symptoms require. It is best to follow the doctor's advice and perhaps write down any instructions so they won't be forgotten.

Measles
Chapter 4
A fever, cough, cold symptoms, sore eyes and a rash are symptoms of this disease. Paracetamol decreases fever and discomfort. Babies are usually immunised against this infectious disease.

Menopause
Chapter 5
A time in a woman's life when periods and child-bearing cease. The average age is late forties or early fifties. About three-quarters of women experience hot flushes and other changes. Hormones are often prescribed.

Middle-ear infections
Chapter 4
The majority of these infections occur in children under ten years of age. They occur frequently because the passageways between ear, nose and throat are not fully developed in children. Treatment usually requires an antibiotic and pain relief.

Migraines
Chapter 2
Migraine headaches are more common in women, and often associated with nausea and vomiting or a visual 'aura'. The usual approach is to try a particular medication, moving on to others if this does not work. Simple analgesics, combined with rest in a darkened room are often effective treatment.

Moles and blemishes
Chapter 3
If moles become itchy or darken, bleed or grow, then advice must be sought from a doctor. These moles may become malignant and early treatment is essential.

Blemishes include port wine stain, fine red lines or capillaries found on the cheeks or nose, birthmarks and some leg veins.

Molluscum contagiosum
Chapter 4
The infection occurs as a crop of pearly to pink raised lesions in the upper part of the body or even on the face which eventually dry up and disappear.

Morning sickness
Chapter 7
A cup of tea, dry biscuits and toast in bed before rising and a large number of small meals can help this condition.

Mumps
Chapter 4
This is a common childhood infection. There is a danger of sterility should it be caught by

adolescent boys or men. Headache, fever and painful swelling of the salivary glands can be treated with pain and fever relief, rest and fluids.

N

'Natural' remedies
Chapter 1
In reality, natural healing is providing the optimum environment for healing to take place. This involves avoiding smoking, alcohol and stress, having a healthy balanced diet, adequate sleep and relaxation.

Nose job or rhinoplasty
Chapter 3
The aim of surgeons now is to produce a more natural looking nose. Before the operation the surgeon should discuss with you the kind of nose you prefer, its attainability and whether it suits your face. Chin surgery sometimes accompanies nose surgery.

O

Obesity
Chapter 1
'Fad' diets only result in short-term weight loss. Healthy eating habits and a sensible exercise program are the answer to obesity. Some people benefit from a support group while losing weight.

Orchitis
Chapter 6
Bacteria and viruses can cause this inflammation of the testis. Mumps orchitis can cause infertility in men.

Osteoporosis
Chapter 5
This is a condition where bones become porous and more able to be broken. About one-quarter of menopausal women will develop osteoporosis due to a fall in hormone levels. It is wise to discuss this condition with your doctor before beginning treatment.

Oestrogen
Chapter 5
This is a naturally occurring female hormone produced by the ovaries, during a woman's reproductive period. Oestrogen can be given as therapy after this time.

P

Periods, absence of
Chapter 5
There is considerable variation in what is the normal time for the onset of menstruation. It is advisable to see your doctor if there has been no period by 15 years of age. If your periods cease and you are not pregnant, see your doctor.

Periods, heavy
Chapter 5
Report any change in bleeding pattern to your doctor. The intrauterine device can cause heavy bleeding. Anaemia can occur if periods are continually heavy.

Periods, painful
Chapter 5
A number of medications are available for severe pain. Doctors can also prescribe the contraceptive Pill to decrease blood flow and diminish pain.

Plantar warts
Chapter 3
Pain occurs if plantar warts develop on the weight-bearing part of the foot. As they are caused by a virus, they may eventually disappear. They can be burnt off with chemical treatments, by freezing or surgery.

Plastic or cosmetic surgery
Chapter 3
There has been increased demand for cosmetic surgery. It can be painful and expensive and complications can occur. It is important the prospective patient has a realistic understanding of what can be achieved and at what cost.

Poisoning
Chapter 2
Swallowing poison accounts for most cases of poisoning, but poison can be inhaled or even absorbed through the skin. Prevention is most important, especially with young children. If poisoning occurs, it is vital not to panic. Contact a doctor or a poisons information centre immediately. Remember to take with you the container with any left-over substance.

Premature ejaculation
Chapter 6
Anxiety, lack of knowledge and

inexperience may contribute to this problem. It is important for a doctor to look for physical factors or emotional problems that could be responsible. Sexual problems and relationship problems may be helped by sexual counselling.

Premenstrual tension (PMT)
Chapter 5
Many women experience symptoms that can be physical, (such as breast discomfort, a feeling of being bloated) or psychological, (such as anxiety, depression, irritability). Symptoms should cease with menstrual flow. Paying attention to stress factors in your lifestyle can be helpful.

Prolapse of the uterus
Chapter 5
If the uterus falls a little in relation to the surrounding tissue, an unpleasant dragging sensation often accompanied by bladder or bowel symptoms can occur

Prostate, enlarged
Chapter 6
The prostate can become enlarged as men get older. Symptoms of enlargement are frequent urination, a urine stream that is slow to start or occurrence of dribbling. If symptoms are severe, the prostate is removed.

Prostatitis
Chapter 6
The prostate gland becomes inflamed due to a bacterial infection. Symptoms include a frequent desire to urinate, urine with an unpleasant odour or showing presence of blood, fever or back pain. Treatment includes administration of antibiotics and an adequate intake of fluid.

R

Relaxation
Chapter 7
Learning self-relaxation techniques is very beneficial to help you lower stress. Healthy leisure activities and regular holidays are also desirable.

Retroverted uterus
Chapter 5
If the uterus is rotated backwards it is known as retroversion and if rotated forward, anteversion.

Roseola
Chapter 4
This viral illness causes a fever and rash in children, generally younger than two years. Treatment is directed towards lowering fever and discomfort.

S

Scoliosis
Chapter 3
A lateral or sideways curve of the spine that develops mostly in girls, in early adolescence. Its cause is unknown, but only a small number of people require treatment consisting of a spinal brace or, rarely, surgery.

Sex, frequency and quality
Chapter 6
There is no strictly defined 'norm' in sexual frequency as long as both partners are satisfied and happy with the number of times they make love. The need for orgasm is varied. Some people experience a satisfying sexual relationship without orgasm. It is essential to communicate with your partner about what pleases you.

Shortsightedness (myopia)
Chapter 3
Both shortsightedness and longsightedness (hypermetropia) are corrected by glasses. A new operation is available to help treat shortsightedness for a selected group of adults whose shortsightedness falls within strictly-defined criteria.

Sick-building syndrome
Chapter 8
Symptoms of headache, lack of energy, stuffy nose, dry throat and eyes and nausea may be experienced by people who work in sealed air-conditioned buildings. Overheating and lack of ventilation may contribute to this syndrome.

Sinusitis
Chapter 2
Sinusitis can produce another form of headache. This can be diagnosed by a doctor as tenderness over the sinuses. Steam inhalation and nasal sniffing of clean salt water can be helpful in clearing the sinuses. If infection is present, appropriate antibiotics are prescribed by a doctor.

Sleep
Chapter 1
There is a great variety in the

amount of sleep that different people require.

Sleeping medication and addiction
Chapter 1
Sleeping medications are best avoided. If taken, medications must be stopped gradually under supervision from a doctor.

Smoking
Chapter 1
Health risks of smoking include strokes, cancer, inflammation of the respiratory tract, heart attacks, stomach, cervical and urinary cancer and circulatory problems. Smokers have bad breath, dull skin, spots and blemishes and premature wrinkles round the eyes and mouth. There are programs designed for people who want to stop smoking. A doctor will advise you on what help is available.

Sprains and strains
Chapter 2
A ligamentous strain is when part of the ligament is stretched, whereas a ligamentous sprain means a ligament is torn at the ends. A torn ligament means that it is no longer attached to the bones. The basic treatment is rest, application of ice, use of a bandage and elevation of the affected part. A torn ligament requires surgery.

Squint (lazy eye, strabismus, cast, turn or cross-eye)
Chapter 3
In a child with a squint, the two eyes do not look at the same thing. One or both eyes can be affected.

Early treatment is essential and may involve wearing glasses or a patch, or undergoing an operation to straighten the eyes.

Suction lipectomy
Chapter 3
This is a specialised technique for removing fat deposits. A double chin, the front of the armpits, the lower stomach, the hips and the thighs are the most suitable areas for this type of surgery. This procedure can result in side effects and complications. Proper patient selection is essential.

Sun care
Chapter 3
It is imperative that everyone become aware of the need to protect themselves from the harmful rays of the sun. Skin cancer related to sun exposure is on the increase. Hats and creams should be used outdoors and solariums avoided. More minor harmful effects of the sun are blemishes and earlier ageing of the skin.

T

Testes, torsion of
Chapter 6
This is a painful condition describing a testis that has become twisted. Shock can develop and an emergency operation will be required to disentangle the torsion.

Testicle, undescended
Chapter 6
A condition in which one or both testes have not fully completed their descent to the scrotal cavity. Treatment involves hormones and sometimes surgery.

Tetanus
Chapter 4
This disease can occur at any age and can cause death. Wounds most likely to result in tetanus include fractured bones where the skin has been broken and penetrating wounds where there is foreign matter in the wound. Immunisation and subsequent booster injections provide immunity.

Thrush (monilia or Candida albicans)
Chapter 8
This organism lives quite normally in the mouth, throat, intestine and vagina. When it multiplies it causes a monilia infection.

In the vagina the infection shows as a thick, white discharge causing an itch. The infection may be passed on to your sexual partner. The doctor may advise both partners to be treated, usually by antifungal creams and pessaries.

Toxic shock syndrome
Chapter 5
A rare condition in which a serious infection is caused by toxic substances released by bacterial infection. It is known to be associated with tampon usage, or can occur after delivery of a baby or as a result of infection occurring under wounds. It is suggested that if you use tampons during the day, use pads during the night. Remember to change tampons frequently and observe very careful hygiene.

Tranquillisers, minor
Chapter 2
The most commonly prescribed

are from the benzodiazepine group of drugs. They are mainly prescribed to treat anxiety and should generally be used only for short periods of time.

Trichomonas
Chapter 8
Trichomonas vaginalis causes this vaginal infection during or just after menstruation. It is characterised by a thin greenish-white discharge with a foul odour. Men can become infected too. Antibiotics are commonly used to treat this condition.

U

Ultrasound
Chapter 1
This procedure involves obtaining an image of the organ by using high frequency sound waves. It is a technique often used in pregnancy. An abdominal ultrasound is often used to detect gall-stones.

Urinary infections
Chapter 8
Women are more prone to these infections, such as cystitis, urethritis, lower urinary tract infection or UTI. The infection is characterised by a burning sensation when urinating, with a frequent desire to urinate. Blood may be present in the urine. It is usual to prescribe an antibiotic. It is important when this infection is present in children to make sure there is no developmental abnormality that could lead to kidney disease.

V

Vaccination
Chapter 4
Routine immunisation has reduced the incidence of certain diseases considerably. Side effects, sometimes serious, can occur. However, the chances of contracting the disease and suffering serious complications are far greater. Illnesses which can be prevented by immunisation include diphtheria, tetanus, whooping cough, polio, measles, mumps, German measles, hepatitis B and Haemophilus influenza.

Vaginismus
Chapter 5
Sometimes inflammation or other conditions can cause the muscles around the vagina to go into spasm. Often emotional reasons underlie this condition. Sexual counselling or a supervised program of gentle stimulation can help.

Varicose and spider veins
Chapter 3
Varicose veins are stretched, enlarged veins caused by blood pooling in them. The valves that control the blood flow in the veins are not working effectively.

Spider veins occur as small purple veins in clusters under the skin. Spending long periods of time standing can promote their development. There are exercises to reverse blood flow in the veins. Treatment includes injections of chemical substances and bandaging, support stockings or sometimes surgical removal of varicose veins.

Vitamins
Chapter 1
Extra vitamins are unneccessary if you have a balanced diet, unless you have a deficiency disease. A placebo or 'dummy pill' often gives the same improvement. As a placebo, therefore, low dose vitamin intake may do some good. Take care with vitamins. Problems can arise with overdosage.

W

Warts
Chapter 3
These unsightly blemishes are a type of viral infection. They may be burnt off surgically or with paints, but if left alone warts will usually disappear.

Weight loss
Chapter 1
Unexplained weight loss, not related to dieting, must be taken seriously. The doctor will look for a cause which can include emotional depression, eating disorders or chronic disease. In the elderly, weight loss can be caused by the side effects of certain types of medications.

INDEX